ANTI-INFLAMMATORY KETO COOKBOOK

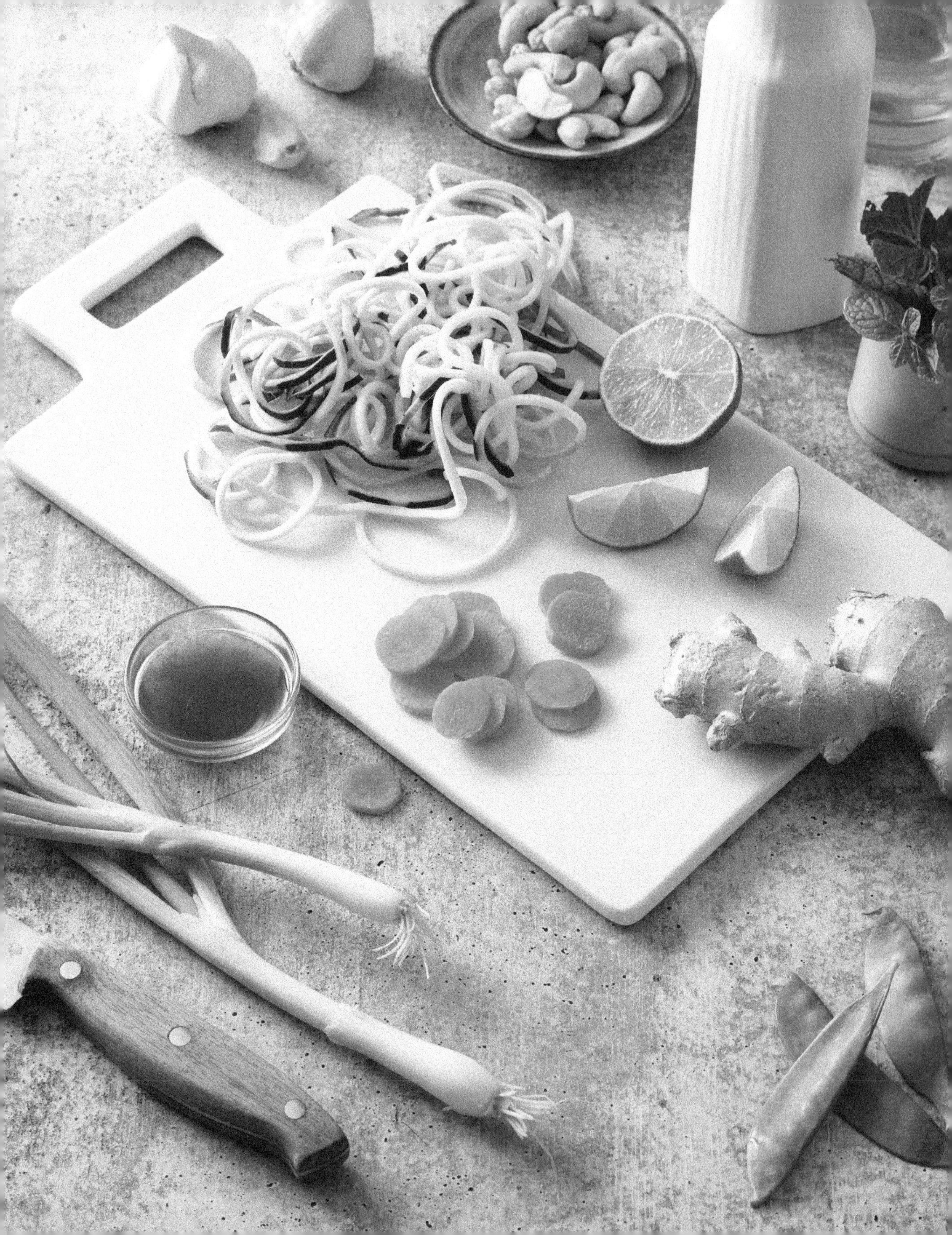

ANTI-INFLAMMATORY KETO COOKBOOK

100 RECIPES AND A 2-WEEK PLAN TO JUMP-START YOUR HEALING

Molly Devine, RD

Photography by Laura Flippen

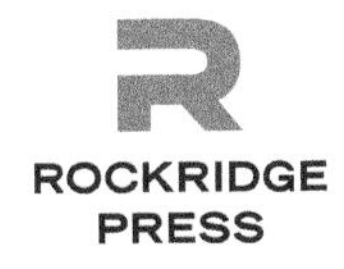

ROCKRIDGE
PRESS

For general information on our other products and services or to obtain technical support, please contact our Customer Care Department within the United States at (866) 744-2665, or outside the United States at (510) 253-0500.

Rockridge Press publishes its books in a variety of electronic and print formats. Some content that appears in print may not be available in electronic books, and vice versa.

Interior and Cover Designer: Lindsey Dekker
Art Producer: Sue Bischofberger
Editor: Anne Lowrey
Production Editor: Rachel Taenzler
Photography © 2020 Laura Flippen
Author photo courtesy of Heba Salama Photography

ISBN: Print 978-1-64739-962-7 | eBook 978-1-64739-963-4
R0

For my family,
who always loves a good meal!

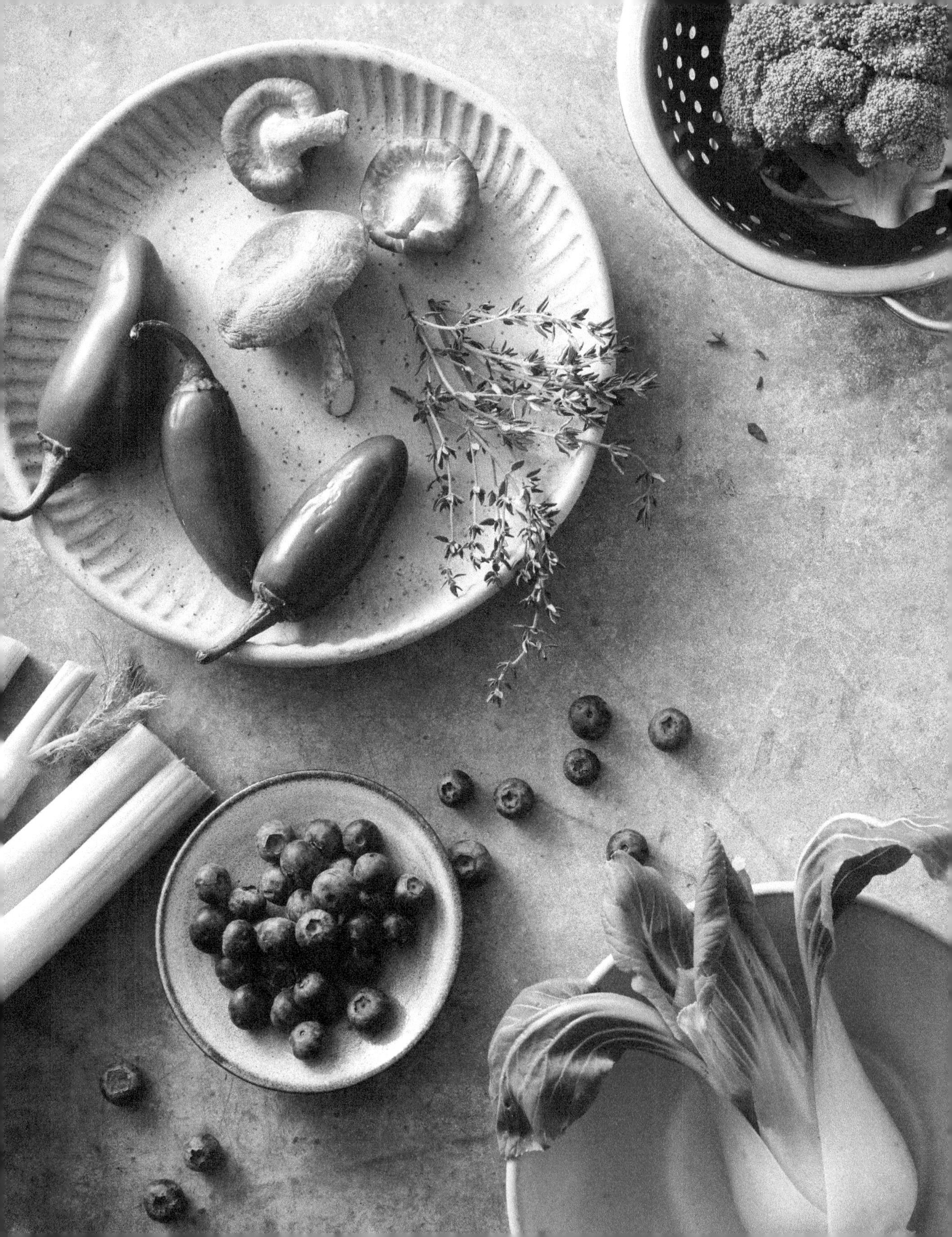

CONTENTS

INTRODUCTION

As a registered dietitian specializing in integrative and functional nutrition, I believe that poor diet and lifestyle practices are the root cause of many chronic diseases and conditions. In many cases, these conditions are entirely preventable by making the necessary nutrition and lifestyle changes that can reverse disease risk early on or drastically reduce symptoms after diagnosis. Rather than simply Band-Aiding a chronic disease or condition with prescriptive medications, we should look at addressing the root of the problem. We can begin to heal the body inside out with medical nutrition therapy, allowing people to improve their health and reverse disease as opposed to simply managing symptoms and accepting a lifelong fate. Food is the best preventive medicine we have available today.

While my nutrition-counseling patients may come to me from different backgrounds and have differing medical diagnoses, they share a common goal to feel better, live longer, and find a sustainable nutrition plan that supports their lifestyle. I believe that most share the same common widespread systemic inflammation. It may manifest itself in various ways, but all can be reduced by the same intervention: dietary and lifestyle changes to reduce inflammation.

I discovered firsthand how following a well-formulated and balanced ketogenic diet can reduce systemic inflammation. As someone with Hashimoto's thyroiditis, an autoimmune hypothyroid condition, I am more susceptible to chronic inflammation. I started to see increased issues with my digestion and gut health, as well as joint pain and injury (which made my regular running and swimming routine suffer). Despite a clean "healthy" diet, I was still seeing symptoms of inflammation on a regular basis.

Following a high-fat/low-carbohydrate ketogenic way of eating brought almost immediate relief from these symptoms, and I was excited to try this approach with my patients. Through my years of employing dietary intervention to achieve and sustain healthy weight, prevent and reverse chronic disease, and improve quality of life, I have no doubt that following a properly formulated ketogenic diet reduces inflammation. It also results in sustainable improvement in overall health.

Not all ketogenic diets are created equal. I don't believe that all are sustainable, nor that they all promote good health. Looking only at macronutrient composition of foods doesn't present a comprehensive view. In this book, I want to help you understand how to create a balanced, varied, and enjoyable ketogenic nutrition approach filled with anti-inflammatory superfoods that will help heal you from the inside out.

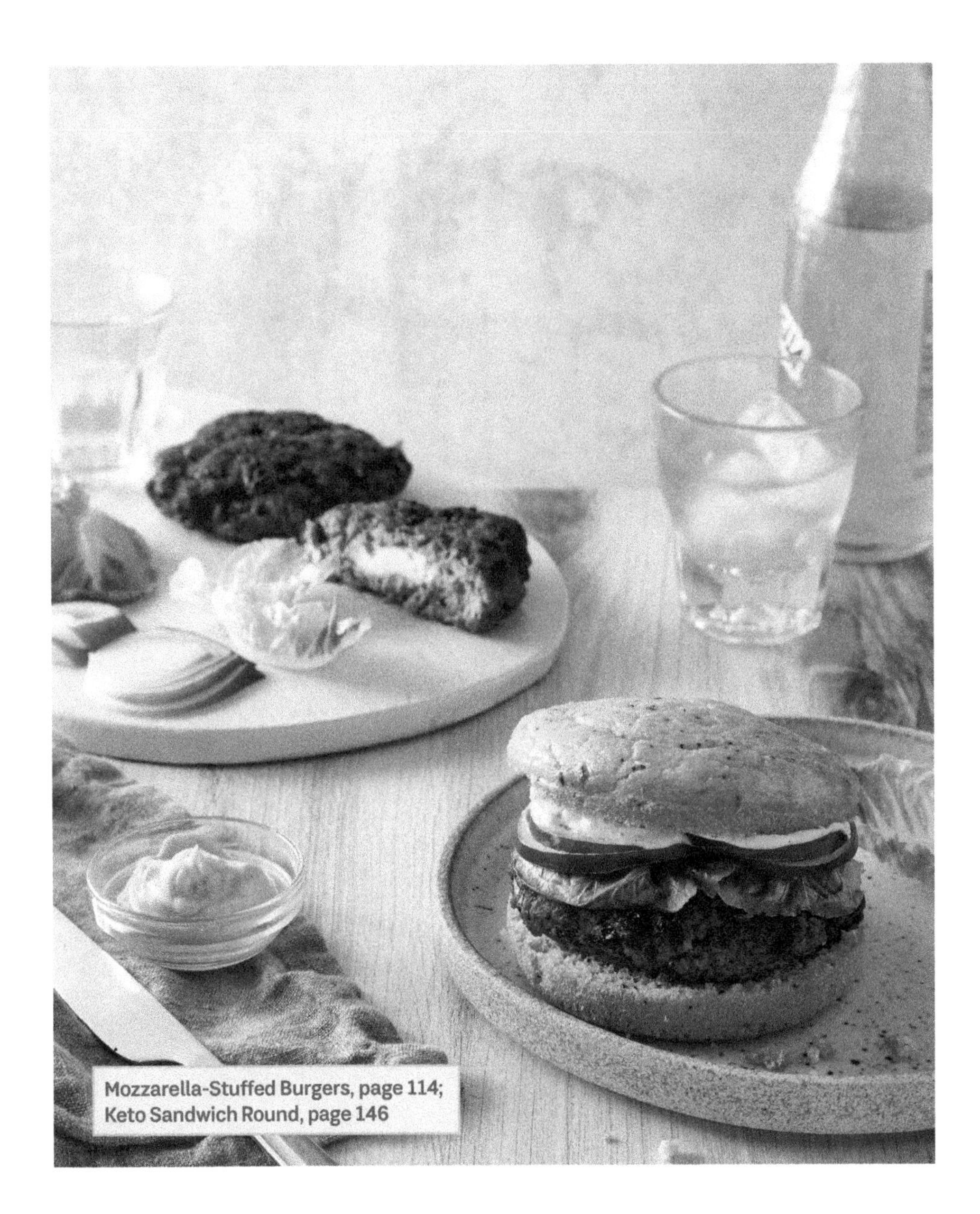
Mozzarella-Stuffed Burgers, page 114;
Keto Sandwich Round, page 146

Food should taste good! Your health and nutrition goals need to align with your expectations for appealing, tasty, and enjoyable foods for any lifestyle change to be sustainable. I hope to appeal to both the novice cook as well as the seasoned chef, and I desire that you find this way of eating and lifestyle to be pleasurable, sustainable, and rewarding.

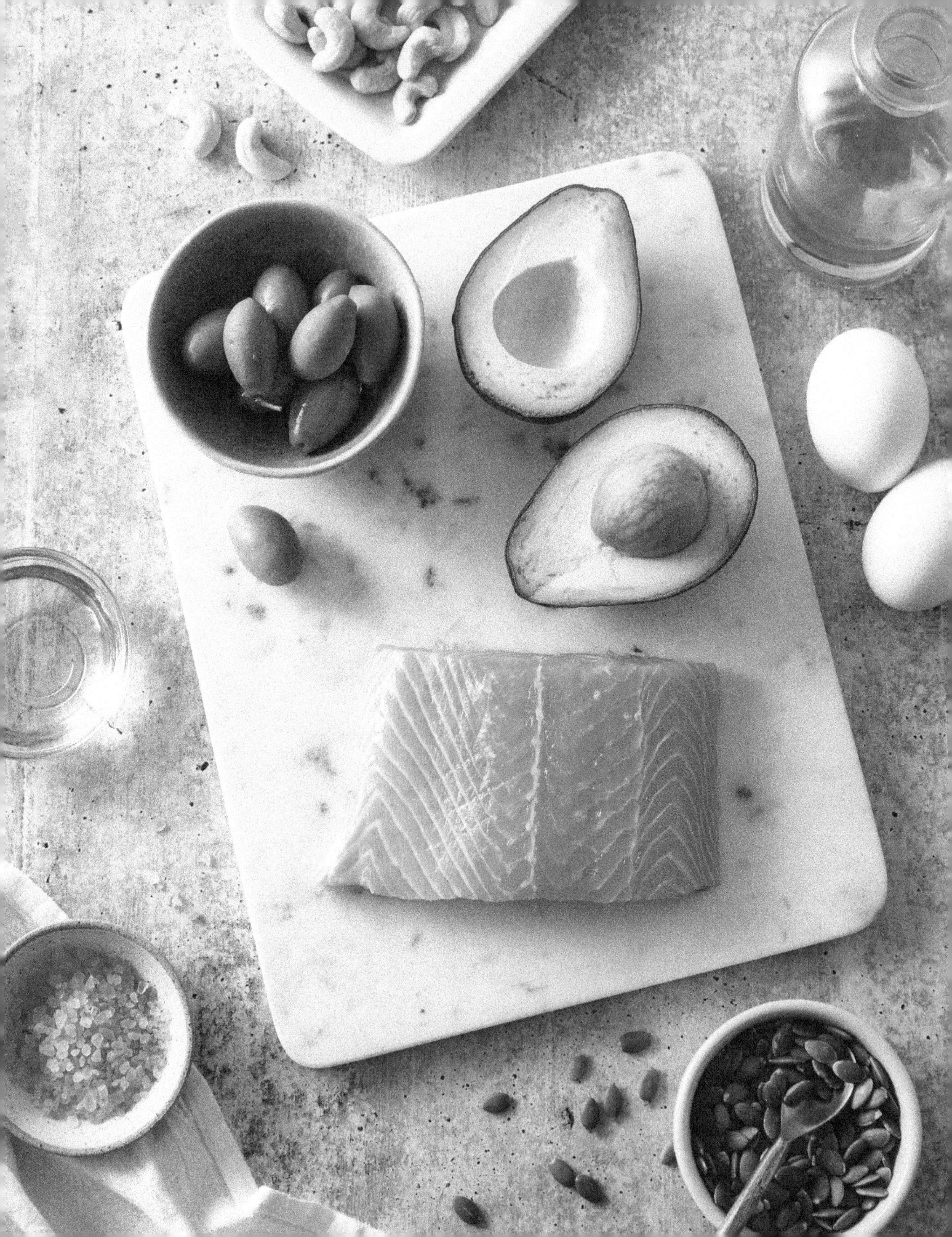

CHAPTER ONE

The Keto Anti-Inflammatory Connection

The ketogenic diet has become more widespread in recent years, mainly due to its effectiveness for substantial weight loss without a focus on caloric restriction and while allowing for rich, satiating foods. While weight loss is a goal (or welcomed side effect) for many, I view it as more of a positive result of a healthy lifestyle change. I encourage my patients to focus instead on the day-to-day improvements in the way they feel. Increased energy, improved mood, decreased joint pain, increased mobility, clearer skin, and reduction in food cravings are all tangible results of reducing inflammation in the body with keto.

In this chapter, I will explain the keto anti-inflammatory connection and help you understand how this way of eating can reduce chronic inflammation and reverse many of its negative side effects, including chronic disease.

UNDERSTANDING INFLAMMATORY RESPONSE

Although we have come to associate the term *inflammation* with negative outcomes, the human inflammatory response is a natural protective action taken by the immune system due to infection, physical stress, trauma, toxic exposure, and short-term illness. It allows our bodies to heal and restore homeostasis, or optimal health and balance.

THE ROLE OF INFLAMMATION IN THE BODY

Acute, or short-term, inflammation is a healthy part of the body's natural healing process. Chronic inflammation, on the other hand, has become more prevalent due to long-term exposure to foods and environmental toxins that cause an inflammatory response. High physical and emotional stress conditions, poor sleep, sedentary lifestyle, and prolonged periods of overweight or obesity also contribute. When our bodies are chronically in an inflammatory, reactive mode, it can be a root cause of many conditions, including allergies, asthma, cancer, diabetes, autoimmune disease, and some degenerative neurological disorders such as Parkinson's and Alzheimer's.

It is important to remember that while prolonged untreated bouts of acute inflammation can lead to chronic inflammation over time, acute inflammatory responses are not uncommon and are a natural part of healthy active lifestyles. Habits and routines are controllable variables in our lives that impact health. You can prevent and reverse many chronic inflammatory conditions by making impactful lifestyle changes now.

SYMPTOMS OF INFLAMMATION

Inflammation often presents in ways that vary from individual to individual. Symptoms vary depending on the cause, the main area affected, and the duration of a condition. Symptoms of acute inflammation also tend to be easier to identify and only affect a localized area. These include pain and tenderness, swelling or fluid retention (edema), redness or rash, shortness of breath (such as in the case of an allergic reaction), and immobility (such as in the case of injury).

Chronic inflammation may manifest itself in similar ways, but it presents a wider range of symptoms that many people overlook or do not associate with inflammation. These symptoms include brain fog; changes in mood; chronic fatigue and exhaustion; gut dysfunction such as bloating, gas, diarrhea, and/or constipation;

	ACUTE INFLAMMATION	CHRONIC INFLAMMATION
CAUSES	• Short-term illness • Brief exposure to toxins or certain foods • Trauma (such as a fall, puncture wound, or surgery) • Physical stress (such as intense exercise or muscle overexertion)	• Acute inflammatory response that is not addressed and becomes a long-term condition • Decreased immune function • Oxidation of cells through long-term exposure to toxic foods or environmental pollutants • Poor dietary choices resulting in long-term overweight or obesity • Long-term physical or emotional stress and/or lack of sleep
ONSET	Immediate	Prolonged
EXAMPLES	• Allergic reaction to a food or substance • Sprained ankle, muscle tear, or other joint injury • Bruise or abrasion • Sunburn • Poison ivy or insect bite	• Insulin resistance, metabolic syndrome, and resulting type 2 diabetes • Auto-immune conditions, such as lupus and rheumatoid arthritis, that cause the body to attack its own cells • Inflammatory bowel disease (IBD) • Skin conditions such as psoriasis and eczema
DURATION	Less than one month; often less than one day when treated	More than one month and up to several years
COMMON TREATMENTS	• Over-the-counter nonsteroidal anti-inflammatory drugs (NSAIDs) such as aspirin and ibuprofen • Corticosteroids such as topical or oral cortisol • RICE protocol for joint or muscle injury: Rest, Ice, Compression, Elevation	• Anti-inflammatory dietary protocol • Prescription medications to target specific disease states and associated symptoms • Oral naturopathic supplements such as curcumin, fish oil, CBD oil

increased food intolerance; chronic skin rash or acne; weight gain; increased blood pressure; and lack of blood sugar control.

Levels of both acute and chronic inflammation can be identified with a blood test for a C-reactive protein (CRP) biomarker. CRP is an acute inflammatory protein that becomes concentrated at sites of inflammation or in the presence of chronic conditions, such as rheumatoid arthritis, cardiovascular disease, and infection. Very few pharmaceutical drugs prescribed to "treat" chronic conditions will decrease CRP levels, although they may reduce symptoms of the condition. Until the inflammatory response has been extinguished, the disease or condition will never fully be treated, only temporarily silenced by pharmacological interventions.

So many of the symptoms of chronic inflammation are more commonly known by their diagnosed chronic disease. Weight gain = obesity. Increased blood pressure = hypertension. Increased blood sugar or hyperglycemia = prediabetes or diabetes. Gut dysfunction = inflammatory bowel syndrome (IBS). Chronic rash = psoriasis. Mental fog or reduced brain function = early onset Alzheimer's. The role of inflammation in the development and progression of certain types of cancer has also been studied extensively. Results link inflammatory response to 15 to 20 percent of all deaths from cancer worldwide. Rather than diagnose and prescribe, let's look at these conditions for what they are: symptoms of a chronically inflamed body. Once we understand the root causes of these symptoms, we can stop the inflammation and reverse the condition.

STEPS YOU CAN TAKE TO REDUCE INFLAMMATION

The good news is that there are steps you can proactively take to lower inflammation in the body and reduce the symptoms of chronic inflammation. From adding certain foods into your diet to examining lifestyle choices, here are some considerations for putting an anti-inflammatory action plan into place.

DIETARY CHOICES

"You are what you eat," as the common phrase goes. The more we research the effects of certain foods on the body, the more this saying rings true. Unfortunately, the standard American diet (SAD) is filled with processed, high-sugar, chemically laden, and artificially enhanced "fake" foods that are causing too many people to feel miserable on a daily basis. If you bought a new car that you were relying on for safe and reliable transportation for your family and you wanted it to last at least 10 years, would you put watered-down gas in it? Never change the oil? Of course not. So, why wouldn't we treat our bodies with the same care and upkeep we give our cars? If we fuel our bodies with foods that cause more harm than good, how do we expect to function at peak performance?

In recent years, the greater medical community has come to better understand the strong connection between adequate and proper nutrition and reduction in disease and death. We see a strong correlation between the consumption of certain foods and increased rates of disease, as well as the importance of making dietary changes to improve and restore health. We know that diets high in sugars and refined processed carbohydrates lead to increased rates of obesity, diabetes, hypertension, and cardiovascular disease, among other complications. The American Heart Association (AHA) has set limits on daily recommendations for added sugars in the diet, and in 2020, the US Food and Drug Administration (FDA) amended the nutrition label on foods to include added sugars along with the percentage of daily recommendation to help Americans adhere to these guidelines. Most people accept and understand that these foods are "unhealthy," but overlook their connection to inflammation as the reason why.

I have found great success treating my patients with a modified ketogenic dietary protocol, which eliminates many pro-inflammatory foods typically accepted as keto-friendly and includes a wide variety of anti-inflammatory fats, colorful fruits and vegetables, and quality protein sources. By focusing on these foods and greatly reducing the amount of carbohydrates in the diet, my anti-inflammatory ketogenic diet protocol is extremely effective at reducing inflammation and improving health while maintaining nutritional variety, palatability, and sustainability.

LIFESTYLE CHANGES

It's important to look at not only what you eat but also how you're living on a day-to-day basis. Positive habits and routines have the ability to impact inflammation as well.

Sleep

Sleep is not a luxury, but a necessity for proper cell and brain function, blood sugar regulation, healthy weight management, and stable mood. Studies show that inadequate sleep elevates blood sugars regardless of dietary or prescription intervention, which leads to weight gain and insulin resistance. I recommend aiming for six to eight hours of sleep nightly. If going to bed late is your normal habit, aim for bedtime 15 minutes earlier every week until you have naturally changed your schedule and increased sleep time.

Physical Activity

Activity doesn't necessarily mean exercise. If you hate the gym, don't force yourself to go; it will only add to your stress levels! Find an activity that you enjoy, and create a new routine of doing it. Walking with a friend (or solo), biking, swimming, dancing, and stretching are all wonderful forms of physical activity that improve heart health, reduce stress and inflammation, and enhance mood. If movement is new to you, set a goal of 5 to 10 minutes daily and increase from there as desired. The important part is to set the routine and habit rather than focusing on the intensity or duration. Once the routine is ingrained, it will be easy to continue as a lifelong practice.

Stress Reduction

Whether it is physical (intense exercise or a physically demanding job) or emotional (work deadlines, family struggles, financial worries), stressful situations put our bodies into "fight or flight" mode, causing insulin spikes, reduced metabolic rate, and increased blood pressure. When temporary, these natural defense mechanisms do not cause long-term damage, but when stress is chronic, it leads to increased risk for disease from a chronic inflammatory state. In our fast-paced world, it is nearly impossible to avoid stress, but we can work toward helping our bodies mitigate its negative impact. Whether through exercise, meditation, reading, journaling, music, massage, or other relaxing activities, it is important to help your body release and handle everyday stress.

WEIGHT LOSS

Achieving and maintaining a healthy weight has long been associated with positive health outcomes. Not only does having less weight to carry around reduce the stress to our joints, heart, lungs, and other vital organs, we also tend to feel better emotionally, which can have a very positive impact on our lifestyle and nutrition choices.

When the body has an excess of stored macronutrients (more body fat than it needs), it stimulates the release of pro-inflammatory factors into the bloodstream. These cause oxidative stress on cells, which can lead to many conditions, including cancer, insulin resistance, metabolic syndrome, and cardiovascular disease. Reducing excess fat storage through healthy weight loss can stop this inflammatory process and reduce the risk of disease.

FIGHTING INFLAMMATION WITH KETO

A well-formulated ketogenic diet excludes sugars, refined carbohydrates, and processed foods, all of which cause inflammation, insulin resistance, and weight gain. For this reason, many doctors and endocrinologists will recommend a ketogenic diet to help their patients manage diabetes and eliminate the need for medications. Aside from just being low carb, following a keto lifestyle fights inflammation in other ways as well.

WHY EATING KETO LOWERS INFLAMMATION

Including a high level of quality healthy fats in your diet that not only provide satiety but have inherently anti-inflammatory properties on their own has amazing health benefits. While poor-quality processed dietary fats and excess adipose tissue can be pro-inflammatory, our body can create anti-inflammatory mediators that work to turn off inflammation in the body from dietary omega-3 fatty acids such as those found in fish, nuts, and seeds, staples of a clean ketogenic diet.

Another well-studied and proven anti-inflammatory effect of a ketogenic diet is the benefit from the high levels of adenosine. This is a naturally occurring compound in the human body made from the breakdown of adenosine triphosphate (ATP) during metabolism, which is greatly increased in the metabolic state of ketosis. The increased level of adenosine has been shown to have an anticonvulsant effect, which is why the ketogenic diet is so widely adopted as a therapeutic treatment for the prevention of seizures and other neurological conditions and disorders. While many nutrition interventions can bring benefits from the foods they include alone, a ketogenic diet has the added powerful health benefit of transitioning the body into a new metabolic state that is inherently anti-inflammatory.

HOW KETO WORKS

Many people confuse a ketogenic diet with simply being "low carb," but it is more complex than that. The majority of energy, or calories, consumed on a ketogenic diet come from dietary fat, only a moderate amount from protein, and a very low amount from carbohydrates. This allows the body to convert from a "glucose burn" (from the breakdown of carbohydrates) to a "fat burn" (from the breakdown of fatty acids) mode, relying on both dietary fat sources as well as stored body fat for energy. This is the metabolic state of *ketosis*, from which the ketogenic diet derives its name.

When you first begin this way of eating, your body will continue to look for glucose for energy, since glucose is the easiest form of fuel for our bodies to use. Most

SUPPLEMENTS TO BOOST YOUR INFLAMMATION FIGHT

While I am always an advocate of looking to well-balanced meals that include healing superfoods as the best source of medical nutrition therapy, there are certain supplements that I do recommend to my patients who have certain dietary restrictions and/or need additional support.

Curcumin (an active component of turmeric). The most widely studied nutrition supplement for natural anti-inflammatory intervention, curcumin is known to possess antioxidant, antibacterial, anticancer, antifungal, and antiviral functions. I love including turmeric, a component in curry powder and fragrant spice blends, in cooking, but the amount needed to see therapeutic benefits greatly exceeds what we are able to ingest from meals alone. Therefore, I advocate supplementing with curcumin capsules for maximum benefit.

Tart cherry juice capsules. Tart cherries have powerful antioxidant properties that help fight off free radicals that cause cell oxidation and damage, but they need to be consumed in high volume to really see the anti-inflammatory benefits. They also contain high amounts of natural sugars that don't align with a ketogenic approach, making concentrated tart cherry powder capsules a wonderful option.

Electrolytes. The four essential electrolytes to focus on are sodium, potassium, calcium, and magnesium. While there are many quality food sources for these in the recipes in this book, I do recommend supplementing with high-sodium broth or an over-the-counter magnesium supplement if muscle soreness, constipation, headache, or other signs of dehydration persist.

Resveratrol. Found in the skin of grapes, this polyphenol has been recognized in numerous studies to contain anti-inflammatory and immune-boosting properties. This is the main reason moderate red wine consumption has been accepted to be a part of a healthy diet and lifestyle. However, the levels of resveratrol that need to be consumed to see therapeutic benefit exceed the amount of red wine that can be safely consumed on a daily basis. Additionally, the alcohol that is present in wine along with this healthy polyphenol has a pro-inflammatory effect on the body. For this reason, I only recommend consuming resveratrol in supplement form to help reduce inflammation.

Alpha-lipoic acid (ALA). This antioxidant is made naturally in the body and found in every cell. It plays vital roles in metabolism and energy production, and its antioxidant properties help reduce inflammation by decreasing cell damage and increasing immunity. It has also been studied as an intervention in preventing cancer. While your body makes ALA on its own, supplementing through capsule form increases levels and boosts its effectiveness.

Fish oil (omega-3s). The essential omega-3 fatty acids eicosapentaenoic acid (EPA) and docosahexaenoic acid (DHA) cannot be synthesized by the body and must be supplemented through the diet. Fatty fish such as wild-caught salmon, mackerel, sardines, and anchovies are excellent sources of these anti-inflammatory powerhouses. I recommend including seafood in your diet three to four times a week. If you are unable to include food sources of EPA and DHA in your diet, I always recommend a fish oil or omega-3 supplement that includes both EPA and DHA.

Cinnamaldehyde. The active component in cinnamon, cinnamaldehyde has also been widely studied and shown to have anti-inflammatory, antioxidant, antitumor, cholesterol-lowering, blood sugar–lowering, and immune-boosting properties. While cinnamon is a delicious and common spice, like turmeric, it is nearly impossible to get the dosage needed for therapeutic benefit from food alone. I recommend supplementing with cinnamon capsules for full benefit.

MCT oil. Medium-chain triglycerides (MCTs) have long been used as a medical nutrition therapy to help those with small intestine dysfunction or malabsorption. Due to the unique length of this fatty acid, it is absorbed differently in our digestive tract, allowing for immediate conversion to ketones for use as energy rather than storage in fat cells. The rapid increase in ketone levels helps with energy, mental clarity, and satiety, deepening the effects of ketosis as an anti-inflammatory metabolic process.

people have two to three days' worth of stored glucose in the form of glycogen, and their bodies will begin the process of breaking down this storage for energy within the first day. Each molecule of glycogen is really one glucose molecule with a few water molecules attached, so as we liberate the glucose to send to our cells for energy, we release stored water along with it.

Water weight loss helps reduce joint stiffness and bloating and produces a result on the scale, but the quick dumping of stored fluid can lead to dehydration from a loss of electrolytes along with the water. Many people talk about experiencing a "keto flu" when trying a ketogenic diet for the first time. However, symptoms of "keto flu" are the same as clinical dehydration and can easily be avoided by sufficient water intake. I recommend drinking half of your body weight in ounces every day (that is, if you weigh 200 pounds, you need to aim for 100 ounces of water daily) and supplementing with essential electrolytes such as sodium, potassium, magnesium, and calcium.

Once your body has depleted most of its glycogen storage, it will need to look for a new fuel source to power the body and brain. Not all cells can use pure fatty acids for fuel, and most important, the brain cannot use them at all. Ketosis is the body's process of converting these fatty acids into usable currency for energy: a ketone. Fatty acids travel to the liver, where they are converted into ketones and sent throughout the body for use as energy. Ketones are like rocket fuel; they are extremely efficient, provide long-term energy, and improve function.

As your body starts to become more and more efficient at the production and use of ketones as its primary fuel source, you can expect a reduction in hunger, improvement in energy, increased mental clarity, improved sleep, and a reduction in inflammation.

OTHER BENEFITS

People come to the ketogenic diet for not just weight loss or anti-inflammatory concerns but also other health benefits. Here are a few to note.

Blood sugar control. Studies show a ketogenic diet can reduce blood sugar and insulin fluctuations due to reduced carbohydrate consumption. Better insulin control and reversing insulin resistance can help improve the associated metabolic disorders, as well as symptoms linked to high insulin and blood sugar, such as type 2 diabetes.

Improved cognitive function, energy, and mood. Aside from the positive psychological associations with improvements in health and physical function, there is science behind the powers of a ketogenic diet on brain health. When the body is in ketosis, the brain utilizes ketones, which leads to feeling more alert and mentally energized throughout the day. The ketogenic diet is currently being studied for its potential beneficial impacts on other neurological diseases, such as Alzheimer's and Parkinson's.

Long-term cardiac health. For decades, we were told that fat will not only make us fat, but that high-fat diets (particularly those high in saturated animal fats) are the main cause for heart disease. We are now learning that this does not represent the full picture. It is the combination of refined and processed carbohydrates and sugars along with a high intake of dietary fats that elevates triglycerides (fat molecules in the blood) and increases the concentration of small particle size LDL cholesterol. Eating a good balance of the right type of "healthy fats" while limiting carbohydrate intake can improve the "good" HDL cholesterol and lower "bad" LDL cholesterol, creating a lower risk for cardiac disease.

INFLAMMATION AND GUT HEALTH

In my practice, patients often come to me for treatment of their irritable bowel syndrome (IBS) and digestive discomfort. Many traditional medical providers use the rather nebulous term *IBS* to diagnose those suffering from a wide range of digestive complications.

Many patients believe that an intolerance to some food or group of foods is the cause of discomfort. I help them understand that, if the gut is inflamed, it is unable to tolerate really *any* food comfortably. When we heal the gut through proper nutrition and lifestyle changes and reduce the inflammatory response, we have restored balance and the body is able to tolerate *all* healthy foods again without pain or complication. I use this as an example of two things: 1) Often chronic inflammation disguises itself as other ailments. In this case, food intolerance. 2) Simply diagnosing a problem without looking for or addressing the root cause of the condition never leads to a solution. We must understand that systemic inflammation can manifest itself in many different ways and once it is addressed and reversed, balance can be restored, and our bodies will function the way they are intended to.

Chaffle and Lox, page 44; Moroccan-Spiced Cauliflower Salad, page 55; Panfried Salmon and Bok Choy in Miso Vinaigrette, page 80; Marinated Antipasto Veggies, page 133

CHAPTER TWO

Eating Keto to Lower Inflammation

So many of the anti-inflammatory benefits derived from following a ketogenic diet stem from the metabolic shift of your body from using glucose to using ketones (from fats) for energy. For this reason, it is important to follow a fairly strict macronutrient profile to allow this process to initiate and continue.

In this chapter, I'll explain what macros are and how to calculate your daily macro needs. I'll introduce the main principles behind the ketogenic diet and the power foods you'll need to begin following an anti-inflammatory keto way of eating.

PLANNING YOUR MACROS

Macronutrients, or *macros* for short, are the building blocks of our diet. All food breaks down into one of three macronutrients—protein, carbohydrate, or fat—and many foods (such as dairy or nuts) are a combination of two or all three. The generally recommended macro ratio for a ketogenic diet is 70 to 75 percent fat, 20 to 25 percent protein, and 5 to 10 percent carbohydrate. However, certain individuals have higher protein needs and/or can tolerate higher levels of carbohydrates from high-fiber, plant-based sources while maintaining ketosis.

High fat (70 to 75 percent of daily calories). Keto enthusiasts love being able to enjoy rich, satiating foods but sometimes overlook the importance of quality fat choices. High fat doesn't mean unlimited bacon, butter, cream, and steak. The most beneficial anti-inflammatory ketogenic diet is rich in heart-healthy unsaturated fats from plant and marine sources and keeps saturated fats from animals at a minimum.

Moderate protein (20 to 25 percent of daily calories). One of the biggest differences between a ketogenic diet and a low-carb/high-protein diet is the moderation of protein. That's because our bodies will turn excess protein (and in small amounts, excess fat) into glucose for use as fuel *before* producing ketones. This process is called *gluconeogenesis* and is a normal daily process, even for those on a ketogenic diet, because glucose is essential for a number of bodily functions. However, when dietary protein is in excess of the body's need on a regular basis, the body will continue to run on glucose, thus preventing ketosis or fat-burn. Most people overconsume protein, thinking that it only goes to their muscles. In fact, most people cannot absorb more than 25 to 35 grams of protein per meal, which amounts to roughly four to six ounces of meat or fish. The excess will get converted into glucose and diminish anti-inflammatory ketogenic progress.

Low carb (under 10 percent of daily calories). I emphasize the importance of plant-based carbohydrates, such as nonstarchy vegetables and low-sugar fruits, rather than processed keto-friendly packaged food products. The former are chock-full of micronutrients (aka vitamins and minerals), which are essential for cell function, metabolism, digestion, and overall health and energy. The latter tends to be mostly "filler fibers" that the body cannot process well, chemicals and additives such as artificial sweeteners and dyes, and inflammatory fats. For this reason, I don't look at "net carbs" (total carb grams minus fiber grams) but rather total carbs as the best number to watch. The carbohydrates in your diet should come from primary plant sources for maximum anti-inflammatory benefits.

CHOOSING YOUR FAT AND PROTEIN SOURCES WISELY

For optimal anti-inflammatory benefit, the majority of the fat calories in your diet should come from omega-9-rich monounsaturated fatty acids (MUFAs), found in foods such as olive and avocado oil, and omega-3-rich polyunsaturated fatty acids (PUFAs), found in foods such as fatty fish and many nuts and seeds. Other PUFAs include omega-6 fatty acids, which can be pro-inflammatory when eaten in excess. Since omega-6 fatty acids are much more prevalent in the standard American diet (SAD), it is important to make an effort to increase your omega-3 fatty acid consumption.

The recipes that follow are full of excellent sources of anti-inflammatory MUFAs and omega-3 fatty acids, such as olive oil, avocados, fatty fish, free-range eggs, nuts, and seeds. Animal proteins can also be great sources of omega-3s, but quality is important. When possible, aim for grass-fed meats and dairy, pasture-raised or free-range poultry, pork, and eggs, and wild-caught seafood. Use mostly olive oil and grass-fed butter (in moderation) when cooking, and avoid processed cooking oils such as canola, corn, and soy. Look out for these in condiments such as mayonnaise and bottled salad dressings, choosing instead to make your own with some of the recipes provided in this book. Avoiding processed and "boxed" foods will largely reduce your omega-6 consumption.

Think of saturated fats as a guest star, not the main attraction. Fattier cuts of red meat and pork, cured meats like bacon and prosciutto, butter and cream, and cheeses lend intense flavor and help boost fat ratios in many meals and keto-friendly treats. Fortunately, a little can go a long way. The recipes in the following chapters will help you better understand this concept while allowing you to include a wide variety of foods into your diet. Note that the dessert recipes may contain higher levels of saturated fats and dairy. Fitting with healthy lifestyle and dietary practices, these should be thought of as treats and kept in moderation or saved for special occasions.

CHOOSING ANTI-INFLAMMATORY KETO FOODS

The following table will help you choose anti-inflammatory foods. I have noted those foods, spices, and herbs that have been studied and shown to have anti-inflammatory properties with an *. I include these in many of the recipes in this book, and I encourage you to add these flavorful components to some of your favorite recipes to boost your immunity and support your anti-inflammatory journey.

	ENJOY	EAT IN MODERATION	AVOID
VEGETABLES	Leafy greens (arugula, kale, radicchio lettuces, spinach); green beans; asparagus; cruciferous vegetables* (broccoli, Brussels sprouts, cauliflower); onions*; fennel*; summer squash (yellow squash and zucchini); bell peppers; celery; mushrooms; eggplant; pickles; garlic*; radish	Carrots; pumpkin and other winter squash; tomatoes	Potatoes; yams; corn; peas
FISH AND SEAFOOD	All, with an emphasis on high-fat, lower-mercury fish, such as wild-caught salmon*, mackerel*, sardines*, and anchovies*	Farm-raised fish (salmon, shrimp, tilapia)	
MEATS AND PROTEINS	Leaner cuts of grass-fed beef and bison; pasture-raised pork; free-range poultry; free-range eggs	Higher-fat cuts of grass-fed beef and lamb, nitrate-free bacon; cured meats like prosciutto and salami	Processed meats like Spam, hot dogs, deli meat

	ENJOY	EAT IN MODERATION	AVOID
DAIRY AND CHEESE	Full-fat goat and sheep's milk cheeses, low-lactose hard cheeses such as Parmesan and Asiago; whole milk Greek or Icelandic yogurt	Cow's milk softer cheeses such as Cheddar and mozzarella; butter; heavy whipping cream; sour cream; full-fat cream cheese (aim for grass-fed when possible)	Sweetened yogurts; milk; processed cheeses such as low-fat or part-skim cheese and cream cheese
GRAINS AND LEGUMES			All, including peanuts
FRUITS	Avocados, dark berries* (blueberries, raspberries, blackberries, strawberries), lemons, limes	Oranges and clementines	Higher-sugar fruits (apples, pears, peaches, plums, cherries, melon)
NUTS, SEEDS, AND FLOURS	All tree nuts and nut butters (coconuts, almonds, Brazil nuts, cashews, filberts/hazelnuts, macadamia nuts, pecans, pine nuts, walnuts); chia, flax, and hemp seeds; pumpkin seeds; sesame seeds and tahini (sesame seed paste)	Almond flour; coconut flour	White flour, whole-wheat flour, chickpea flour, rice flour
FATS AND OILS	Olive oil; olives; avocado oil; avocado mayo; coconut oil and full-fat unsweetened coconut milk; MCT oil	Sesame oil	Processed vegetable oils (canola, corn, soybean)

	ENJOY	EAT IN MODERATION	AVOID
SWEETENERS, SPICES, AND SEASONINGS	Herbs (especially basil*, rosemary*, mint*); unsweetened spices (especially cinnamon*, nutmeg*, clove*, turmeric*, fennel seed*, red pepper flakes*, black pepper*, saffron*); salt; vanilla extract; red wine and apple cider vinegar; stone-ground mustard; unsweetened hot sauce; Worcestershire sauce	Balsamic vinegar; monk fruit; stevia	Sugar of any kind (honey, maple syrup, brown sugar, cane sugar, corn syrup, agave); ketchup; barbecue sauce; seasoning blends that include sugar (cinnamon sugar blend); artificial sweeteners (Splenda, Sweet'N Low); sugar alcohols (erythritol, sorbitol)
BEVERAGES	Water, unsweetened flavored seltzer waters, unsweetened teas (herbal tea, black tea, green tea)	Black coffee; fruit-infused waters; plant-based milks; red wine	Sodas; juices (even 100 percent fruit); beer and spirits; dessert wines; spiked seltzers; cow's milk; sweetened teas and coffee drinks

PREPARING FOR KETO SUCCESS

Making lifestyle changes and changing the way you eat can feel overwhelming at first. The tips in this section will help you successfully start off your anti-inflammatory ketogenic lifestyle on the right foot.

Don't go hungry. Even if you do have a weight loss goal, a ketogenic diet does not rely on caloric restriction for success. Rather, it focuses on the type and quality of food in your meals. Your main goal in the first few weeks is to transition your body into ketosis and avoid the foods that cause inflammation. Your body will naturally adjust to this new way of eating. Cravings will lessen and natural satiety will dominate, but in the first few weeks, don't worry about how many snacks you may need to include during the day to get over the "hump," so long as these foods fall within the guidelines outlined in this chapter.

Attack carb or sugar cravings with fat. If you have a craving for something carb-heavy, attack it with a fatty snack, such as those listed in chapter 9 (see page 131). Think of this as retraining the brain from searching for glucose for energy to learning to utilize ketones made from the breakdown of fatty acids. Be sure to have plenty of convenient, satisfying snacks and meals on hand to avoid giving in to a craving.

Create a new routine. For many, poor dietary choices are simply the result of unhealthy routines that can be hard to break out of, whether that is grabbing a sweet treat after dinner, eating in front of a screen, or sitting on the couch as soon as you walk through the door at the end of a long day. It's hard to just give up these habits without replacing them with a new routine. Make a mug of herbal tea after dinner instead of a dessert, eat meals at a table and free of distractions, or take a 5- to 10-minute walk to decompress at the end of your day.

Be kind to yourself. You are not a robot and you are not perfect. Make sure to give your body what it needs to be successful. Get adequate sleep, aiming for six to eight hours. Don't overdo it with exercise—you may need to cut back on intensity or duration of your current physical activity routine until your body has adjusted. Sticking to your meal plan and nutrition goals is the most important part of starting this anti-inflammatory lifestyle.

STOCKING YOUR REFRIGERATOR AND PANTRY

A well-stocked refrigerator, freezer, and pantry can make meal preparation and nutrition compliance so much easier! The following list is a great starting point with many of the staple ingredients found in the recipes that follow.

Pantry Basics

- Broth or stock: chicken, beef, or vegetable
- Canned full-fat coconut milk
- Canned seafood: tuna, salmon, mackerel
- Canned tomatoes: paste, diced, and pureed (no sugar added)
- Nuts: almonds, walnuts, pecans, macadamia nuts, hazelnuts, Brazil nuts, pistachios

- Oils: avocado, coconut, olive
- Seeds: flaxseed, chia, pumpkin, sesame
- Spices: cinnamon, cloves, nutmeg, ground ginger, turmeric, red pepper flakes, fennel seed, cumin, garlic powder, onion powder, curry powder
- Teas: herbal, black, and green (no sugar added)
- Unsweetened (artificially or naturally) seltzer waters
- Unsweetened nut and seed butters: almond, sunflower, and tahini (sesame seed paste)
- Vinegar: apple cider, red wine, white wine, rice

Refrigerator and Freezer Basics

- Avocados (store unripe avocados in a dark place at room temperature; store ripe avocados in the refrigerator so that they last longer)
- Butter: grass-fed
- Cheeses of quality: goat cheese, feta (preferably from sheep's milk), Parmesan, and grass-fed cow's milk cheeses such as Cheddar and mozzarella
- Citrus: lime and lemon
- Eggs: preferably free-range for the best-quality fats
- Frozen berries: strawberries, blueberries, raspberries, and blackberries
- Frozen veggies: broccoli, spinach/greens, green beans, asparagus, Brussels sprouts, bell peppers, cauliflower, riced cauliflower, and green and yellow squash (avoid vegetable blends containing peas, corn, beans, potatoes, and mushrooms)
- Mayo of quality: made with avocado or olive oil or homemade Anti-Inflammatory Mayo (page 148)
- Salad greens: arugula, spinach, kale, baby lettuces, romaine, and mixed greens
- Veggies: cucumber, bell pepper, cherry tomatoes, celery, broccoli, cauliflower, radishes, and carrots
- Whole milk Greek yogurt

SETTING UP YOUR KITCHEN

You don't have to be a professional chef or have a state-of-the-art kitchen to prepare ketogenic meals, but having the following tools will make it all come together faster. I've broken these down into two lists: basic tools that should be found in most kitchens and "nice to have" items that will help save on pricey store-bought prepped ingredients.

Basic Tools

Cutting boards. Wood, composite, or synthetic are all fine, depending on your preference.

Garlic press. This simple tool helps impart great garlic flavor into sauces, dips, and dressings without the harshness of larger garlic pieces.

Glass baking dishes. A 9-by-13-inch and an 8-inch-square are used in many of the recipes and can double as storage for leftovers as well.

Measuring cups and spoons. I recommend cups ranging from ¼ to 1 cup and spoons from ⅛ of a teaspoon up to 1 tablespoon.

Roasting pans and/or baking sheets. There is no need to invest in expensive baking sheets. I favor lining mine with either aluminum foil or parchment paper before using to minimize cleaning time.

Saucepans and skillets. A variety of sizes will work. If you will be doubling any of the recipes for leftovers or to enjoy with friends and family, you will want to have larger pots and pans for cooking. I love a 10- to 12-inch cast-iron skillet for searing fish and meats, but a regular medium skillet will be just fine.

Sharp knives. The knife is the most important tool for any chef and quality sharp knives can help prevent kitchen accidents and make meal prep a breeze.

Whisk. A simple medium-size whisk will help make sauces smooth and eggs fluffy.

Nice to Have

Box grater and zester. These are the best ways to create fresh flavor and added nutrition from citrus zest, grated cheese, and even shredded veggies.

Food processor. This is definitely a little more of an investment, but as the keto way of eating truly becomes a lifestyle, the monetary and time savings from homemade riced cauliflower, finely slivered or chopped vegetables, pesto, dressings, sauces, and homemade nut butters will certainly pay off.

Immersion blender or stand blender. Great for making smoothies, dressings, sauces, and soups. I prefer an immersion blender because it is affordable, versatile, and easy to clean.

Spiralizer. This is a wonderful addition to a low-carb kitchen! Many grocery stores now offer prepared spiralized veggies in the refrigerated produce section, but spending two minutes making these yourself will save you money in the long run.

MEAL PLANS

The best way to turn diet intention into diet reality is to plan and prep meals ahead of time. I have designed a two-week meal plan that includes three daily meals to fit the ideal macronutrient ratios. These set you up for a successful transition into ketosis using a variety of the delicious recipes found in this book.

You can adjust the amount of cooking to fit your needs and preferences. I've included some leftovers to minimize your time spent cooking. Do what works best for you. You'll find a shopping list for each week to include all the ingredients you will need to make the recipes for that week (excluding the snack ideas). If you decide to double up recipes and omit others to save on cooking time, you will need to modify these shopping lists.

Snack options are included, and most can be made ahead on the weekend, but they are there only if you feel hunger between meals. Typically, snacks are helpful during the first week, as your body has not fully transitioned into ketosis and may continue to crave the constant stream of energy it was getting from glucose. However, as your body adjusts to burning fat for fuel, it begins to reduce cravings for carbohydrates and relies on stored body fat for energy between meals. At this point, you will likely begin to feel more satiety and less need for snacking, which is a great sign your body is making a metabolic shift. If you do not feel the need for the snacks, by all means do not include them.

WEEK 1 MENU

	MONDAY	TUESDAY	WEDNESDAY	THURSDAY	FRIDAY	SATURDAY	SUNDAY
BREAKFAST	Pumpkin Pie Yogurt Bowl (page 39)	Tofu and Veggie Scramble (page 40)	***Leftover*** Tofu and Veggie Scramble	Blueberry Smoothie with Lemon and Ginger (page 42)	Pumpkin Pie Yogurt Bowl (page 39)	Cherry-Coconut Pancakes (page 38)	Salmon Cakes Benedict with Lemon-Turmeric Aioli (page 34)
LUNCH	Lemony Chicken Salad with Blueberries and Fennel (page 48) over 2 cups mixed greens	***Leftover*** Panfried Salmon and Bok Choy in Miso Vinaigrette	***Leftover*** Lemony Chicken Salad with Blueberries and Fennel in a Keto Sandwich Round (page 146)	Weekday Omega-3 Salad (page 58)	***Leftover*** Chicken Margherita	Salmon Salad Sushi Bites (page 138)	Turmeric and Avocado Egg Salad (page 74)
DINNER	Panfried Salmon and Bok Choy in Miso Vinaigrette (page 80)	Chicken Margherita (page 104)	Turkey Meatloaf Muffins with Avocado Aioli (page 99)	***Leftover*** Turkey Meatloaf Muffins with 2 cups mixed greens tossed in Creamy Lime-Cilantro Dressing (page 155)	Weeknight Greek Salad (page 60) with 4-ounce can olive oil–packed tuna	Bison Burgers in Lettuce Wraps (page 98)	***Leftover*** Bison Burgers with ***leftover*** Weeknight Greek Salad

SNACK IDEAS

Anti-Inflammatory Power Bites (page 132): Store these in the freezer to have across the two weeks.

Marinated Antipasto Veggies (page 133): You'll use these in the Greek salad.

Pimento Cheese (page 141) and Seedy Crackers (page 139): Double the cracker recipe and store the leftovers in the freezer for week 2.

Matcha Fat Bombs (page 126): Store these in the freezer to have across the two weeks.

WEEK 1 SHOPPING LIST

PRODUCE

- Avocados, ripe (7)
- Baby arugula (16 ounces)
- Baby bok choy (8 heads)
- Basil (1 bunch)
- Bell pepper, red (1)
- Bibb lettuce (1 head)
- Blueberries, fresh or frozen (½ cup)
- Celery stalks (2)
- Cilantro (1 large bunch)
- Cucumbers, large (2)
- Garlic (2 heads)
- Jalapeño (1) (optional)
- Lemons (7)
- Limes (2)
- Mixed greens (1 [5-ounce] bag)
- Mushrooms, small button (1 pint)
- Onion, red (1)
- Oregano (1 bunch)
- Parsley (1 bunch)
- Romaine lettuce (1 large head)
- Rosemary (1 bunch)
- Scallions (1 bunch)
- Sweet peppers, snack-size (8)

SEAFOOD, POULTRY, AND MEAT

- Bison, ground (1 pound)
- Chicken breast (2 pounds)
- Salmon fillet, wild-caught (1½ pounds)
- Turkey, ground (1 pound)

DAIRY, EGGS, AND CHILLED

- Eggs, large (13)
- Feta cheese, sheep's milk (8 ounces)
- Greek yogurt, plain, whole milk (1 [32-ounce] container)
- Heavy whipping cream (1 pint)
- Mozzarella, fresh (4 ounces)
- Tofu, firm (8 ounces)

CANNED AND BOTTLED ITEMS

- Almond milk, unsweetened (1 cup)
- Artichoke hearts (1 [14-ounce] can)
- Olives, pitted black or green (1 [6-ounce] jar)

- **Olives,** pitted Kalamata (1 [6-ounce] jar)
- **Pumpkin puree,** unsweetened (1 [15-ounce] can)
- **Tuna,** olive-oil packed (2 [4-ounce] cans)

FROZEN FOODS

- **Blueberries,** frozen (¼ cup)
- **Dark cherries,** frozen (1 cup)

PANTRY

- **Almond flour**
- **Almond meal**
- **Almonds,** slivered
- **Baking powder**
- **Black pepper,** ground
- **Capers**
- **Cayenne pepper,** ground
- **Cinnamon,** ground
- **Coconut flour**
- **Cumin,** ground
- **Dijon mustard**
- **Fennel seed**
- **Flaxseed,** ground
- **Garlic powder**
- **Ginger,** ground
- **Miso paste**
- **Monk fruit extract or sugar-free sweetener (optional)**
- **Nori seaweed**
- **Oil,** avocado
- **Oil,** coconut
- **Oil,** extra-virgin olive
- **Oil,** sesame
- **Oil,** toasted sesame
- **Oregano,** dried
- **Pecans**
- **Pumpkin pie spice**
- **Pumpkin seeds**
- **Red pepper flakes**
- **Rosemary,** dried
- **Salt**
- **Sesame seeds**
- **Smoked paprika**
- **Sriracha or other hot sauce**
- **Tamari**
- **Tomato paste,** no sugar added
- **Turmeric,** ground
- **Vanilla extract**
- **Vinegar,** rice wine
- **Vinegar,** white

WEEK 2 MENU

	MONDAY	TUESDAY	WEDNESDAY	THURSDAY	FRIDAY	SATURDAY	SUNDAY
BREAKFAST	Almond Butter and Cacao Nib Smoothie (page 43)	2 eggs scrambled in 1 tablespoon olive oil, topped with Spiced Guacamole (page 152)	Lemon-Herb Baked Frittata (page 65)	Almond Butter and Cacao Nib Smoothie (page 43)	***Leftover*** Lemon-Herb Baked Frittata	Scrambled Eggs with Mackerel (page 36)	Chaffle and Lox (page 44)
LUNCH	Vegan Creamy Asparagus Soup (page 50) with ***leftover*** Salmon Cakes (from week 1)	***Leftover*** Slow-Cooker Pulled Pork with ***leftover*** Vegan Creamy Asparagus Soup	***Leftover*** Slow-Cooker Pulled Pork and ***leftover*** Classic Coleslaw on a Keto Sandwich Round (page 146)	***Leftover*** Swordfish Kebabs with Mint Cream over 2 cups mixed greens with ***leftover*** Basic Vinaigrette	***Leftover*** Moroccan-Spiced Cauliflower Salad with 4-ounce can olive oil-packed tuna or salmon	***Leftover*** Lemon-Herb Baked Frittata with 2 cups mixed greens with ***leftover*** Basic Vinaigrette	Baked Spiced Tofu (page 71) over ***leftover*** Perfect Riced Cauliflower
DINNER	Slow-Cooker Pulled Pork (page 110) with Classic Coleslaw (page 59)	Swordfish Kebabs with Mint Cream (page 85) and 2 cups mixed greens with Basic Vinaigrette (page 147)	South-western Stuffed Peppers (page 69) with ***leftover*** Spiced Guacamole	***Leftover*** Slow-Cooker Pulled Pork with Moroccan-Spiced Cauliflower Salad (page 55)	***Leftover*** Southwestern Stuffed Peppers with 2 cups mixed greens with ***leftover*** Basic Vinaigrette	Sautéed Shrimp with Arugula Pesto (page 84) over Perfect Riced Cauliflower (page 156) (make ½ batch)	***Leftover*** Sautéed Shrimp with Arugula Pesto tossed with 1½ cups zucchini noodles

SNACK IDEAS

Leftover **Matcha Fat Bombs and Anti-Inflammatory Power Bites from week 1**

Crab and Artichoke Dip (page 134) and Seedy Crackers (page 139)

Loaded Feta (page 135)

OTHER COMBINATIONS:

Almond butter and celery sticks

½ avocado with a drizzle of lime juice and a sprinkle of salt

1 ounce nuts with ¼ cup fresh berries

WEEK 2 SHOPPING LIST

PRODUCE

- Arugula (1 [5-ounce] package)
- Asparagus (1 pound)
- Avocados, ripe (2)
- Baby spinach (1 [5-ounce] package)
- Basil (1 large bunch)
- Bell peppers, any color, large (2)
- Cabbage, green (1 head)
- Cabbage, red (1 head)
- Cauliflower (2 heads)
- Celery stalks (2)
- Cilantro (1 large bunch)
- Cucumber (1)
- Garlic (2 heads)
- Jalapeño (1) (optional)
- Lemons (4)
- Mint (1 large bunch)
- Mixed greens (4 [5-ounce] bags)
- Onion (1)
- Onion, red (1)
- Orange (1)
- Oregano (1 bunch)
- Parsley (1 bunch)
- Rosemary (1 bunch)
- Scallions (1 bunch)
- Tomatoes, Roma (2)
- Zucchini (1)

SEAFOOD, POULTRY, AND MEAT

- Pork loin, boneless, untrimmed (2 pounds)
- Shrimp, wild-caught (1 pound)
- Smoked salmon (4 ounces)
- Swordfish steaks (1 pound)

DAIRY, EGGS, AND CHILLED

- Almond milk, unsweetened (1 pint)
- Eggs, large (18)
- Feta cheese, sheep's milk (1 pound)
- Goat cheese (6 ounces)
- Heavy whipping cream (1 pint)
- Mozzarella cheese, shredded (1 cup)
- Parmesan cheese, shredded (½ cup)
- Tofu, extra-firm (2 [14-ounce] packages)

CANNED ITEMS

- Coconut milk, full-fat (1 [13.5-ounce] can)
- Mackerel, olive-oil packed (1 [4-ounce] can)
- Olives, pitted Kalamata or Spanish green (1 [6-ounce] jar)
- Tuna, olive-oil packed (1 [4-ounce] can)

PANTRY

- Almond butter, unsweetened
- Almond extract (optional)
- Almond flour
- Baking powder
- Black pepper, ground
- Cacao nibs
- Capers

- Chili powder
- Cinnamon, ground
- Cocoa powder, unsweetened
- Cumin, ground
- Dijon mustard
- Everything bagel seasoning
- Garlic powder
- Ginger, ground
- Monk fruit extract or sugar-free sweetener (optional)
- Oil, avocado
- Oil, coconut
- Oil, extra-virgin olive
- Pistachios, shelled
- Pumpkin seeds
- Red pepper flakes
- Rosemary, dried
- Salt
- Smoked paprika
- Tahini
- Turmeric, ground
- Vegetable stock
- Vinegar, red wine
- Vinegar, white
- Vinegar, white wine
- Walnuts

BEYOND THE FIRST TWO WEEKS

I applaud you for making important nutrition changes to improve your health! As your body makes the transition to ketosis, you should start to see notable reductions in inflammation within one to four weeks. I know that change is hard, but keeping your focus on daily improvements in quality of life will help keep you motivated and on track for long-term success. Remember that no one is perfect, and that some days will be better than others. If you have a bad day, put it behind you and get right back to your plan. Oftentimes, we do not get derailed from success by one incident, but rather the snowball effect that is inevitable when we feel our efforts are hopeless.

As you begin to use the recipes and meal plans in this book, you will learn how to build an ideal anti-inflammatory ketogenic plate that follows the correct ratios of macronutrients and will start to feel more comfortable in social or dining-out situations. Most restaurants now offer low-carb or keto-friendly options, which helps somewhat. Your best bet is to order a protein, preferably fish or seafood, along with nonstarchy vegetables or a side salad. You can add healthy fats such as an olive oil–based dressing, guacamole, or a pesto to these. I suggest keeping a small bottle of olive oil with you for drizzling on salads or vegetables, and I recommend that you don't arrive starving. It will be hard to resist chips, breads, and other carb-heavy fillers if you are ravenously hungry! Have a healthy fat snack such as a Matcha Fat Bomb or Anti-Inflammatory Power Bite one to two hours before dining out to help keep a handle on hunger and cravings.

I have included dietary labels with the recipes to help those who have other dietary restrictions. These include Dairy-Free, Egg-Free, Gluten-Free, Nut-Free, and Vegetarian. Always be sure to check the labels of the products you are buying to make sure they align with your restrictions. For example, make sure that gluten-free products indicate that they were processed in a completely gluten-free facility.

Lastly, you will notice that some of the recipes require more ingredients than you may be used to. These were chosen with your optimal health and well-being in mind. The ingredients reflect the best food choices to fuel our bodies, while considering both anti-inflammatory properties and keto macros. Do your best to stick to it . . . it's worth it for how much better you'll feel!

Chaffle and Lox, page 44

CHAPTER THREE

Breakfast and Brunch

SALMON CAKES BENEDICT WITH LEMON-TURMERIC AIOLI

Serves 4 | Prep Time: 10 minutes | Cook Time: 20 minutes | Dairy-Free, Gluten-Free

In this keto-friendly version of a classic brunch dish, I replace the muffin and ham with omega-3 powerhouse salmon cakes loaded with anti-inflammatory spices and top them with a tangy Lemon-Turmeric Aioli, rich in heart-healthy fats. Great for impressing guests, this dish is sure to be a new favorite for weekend brunch.

- 1 (8-ounce) wild-caught salmon fillet, finely chopped, or canned salmon
- 2 tablespoons minced red onion
- 2 tablespoons Anti-Inflammatory Mayo (page 148)
- ⅓ cup almond flour
- 1 teaspoon garlic powder
- 1 teaspoon ground cumin
- 1 teaspoon salt
- ½ teaspoon ground turmeric
- ½ teaspoon freshly ground black pepper
- Grated zest and juice of 1 lime
- ½ cup extra-virgin olive oil, divided
- 4 large eggs

1. In a large bowl, combine the salmon and onion. Add the mayo and mix well.

2. In a small bowl, whisk together the almond flour, garlic powder, cumin, salt, turmeric, and pepper.

3. Add the flour mixture and lime zest and juice to the salmon and mix well.

4. Form the mixture into four patties, about 2 inches in diameter. Let sit for 15 minutes.

5. In a cast-iron skillet, heat 4 tablespoons of olive oil over medium heat. Add the patties and fry for 2 to 3 minutes per side, until they are browned on each side. Cover the skillet, reduce the heat to low, and cook for another 6 to 8 minutes, or until the patties are set in the center. Remove from the skillet and keep warm.

6. In the same skillet, working in two batches, heat 2 tablespoons of olive oil over medium-high heat. Slowly crack two eggs separately into the oil, trying to keep them from touching, and fry for 1 to 3 minutes on each side, depending on desired doneness. For a runnier egg, fry until just set, about 1 minute on each side. Repeat with the remaining 2 tablespoons of olive oil and two eggs.

¼ cup Lemon-Turmeric Aioli (page 149), for serving
Smoked paprika, for serving
Lemon wedges, for serving

7. To serve, top each salmon cake with a fried egg and 1 tablespoon of aioli. Sprinkle with paprika and serve with a lemon wedge.

MAKE AHEAD: These salmon cakes freeze and reheat beautifully, and the aioli will keep in the refrigerator for up to two weeks. Thaw the salmon cakes and reheat in the oven at 350°F for 10 to 15 minutes. Serve topped with a poached or fried egg and leftover aioli or over a mixed green salad with Basic Vinaigrette (page 147).

Per Serving (1 salmon cake, 1 egg, 1 tablespoon aioli): Calories: 645; Total Fat: 61g; Total Carbs: 5g; Net Carbs: 3g; Fiber: 2g; Protein: 22g; Sodium: 816mg;
Macros: Fat: 85%, Carbs: 1%, Protein: 14%

SCRAMBLED EGGS WITH MACKEREL

Serves 4 | Prep Time: 5 minutes | Cook Time: 10 minutes | Gluten-Free, Nut-Free

This is my spin on a classic Jamaican breakfast favorite, ackee and saltfish. Ackee is actually a fruit, native to tropical West Africa, with a nutrition profile similar to that of avocado. When prepared, it is buttery and creamy and resembles scrambled eggs. Canned fatty fish, full of anti-inflammatory omega-3 fatty acids, is perfect for mixing into everyday dishes like this one.

6 large eggs
2 ounces goat cheese, at room temperature
7 tablespoons extra-virgin olive oil, divided
1 teaspoon garlic powder
½ teaspoon freshly ground black pepper
2 Roma tomatoes, finely chopped
2 tablespoons minced onion
1 (4-ounce) can olive oil–packed mackerel, chopped and oil reserved
¼ cup chopped pitted Kalamata or Spanish green olives
2 tablespoons chopped fresh parsley, oregano, rosemary, or cilantro

1. In a small bowl, whisk together the eggs, goat cheese, 2 tablespoons of olive oil, garlic powder, and pepper.

2. In a medium nonstick skillet, heat 1 tablespoon of olive oil over medium-low heat. Add the tomatoes and onion and sauté for 2 to 3 minutes, until they are soft and the water from the tomato has evaporated. Add the egg mixture to the skillet and scramble, stirring constantly with a spatula, for 3 to 4 minutes, until the eggs are set and creamy.

3. Remove the skillet from the heat and stir in the mackerel and reserved oil, olives, and parsley. Serve warm with each serving drizzled with an additional 1 tablespoon of olive oil.

INGREDIENT TIP: Fatty fish such as mackerel, sardines, and anchovies are loaded with inflammation-reducing omega-3 fatty acids but can be intimidating for those that aren't used to eating them. This recipe gives a nice introduction to using these fish in your cooking, but you can substitute canned or smoked salmon for the stronger-tasting mackerel, if preferred.

Per Serving: Calories: 479; Total Fat: 45g; Total Carbs: 4g; Net Carbs: 3g; Fiber: 1g; Protein: 17g; Sodium: 400mg; **Macros:** Fat: 85%, Carbs: 1%, Protein: 14%

COCONUT MILK SMOOTHIE BOWL

Serves 2 | Prep Time: 5 minutes | Dairy-Free, Egg-Free, Gluten-Free

Smoothie bowls are a fun spin on the on-the-go breakfast option, but many are loaded with carbs from the high-sugar add-ins and tropical fruits. This dairy-free keto-friendly version is filling and nutrient dense without packing a sugar punch. The addition of collagen protein powder makes this a well-rounded complete meal that benefits joint, skin, nail, hair, and gut health. Feel free to substitute a protein powder of your choice if you happen to have another on hand.

1 cup full-fat canned coconut milk
½ cup frozen mixed berries
2 scoops unflavored collagen protein powder
2 tablespoons shredded unsweetened coconut
2 tablespoons chia or hemp seeds
2 tablespoons chopped macadamia nuts
Grated lime zest (optional)

1. Place the coconut milk, berries, and protein powder in a blender and process until very smooth.

2. Divide the mixture between bowls. Top each with 1 tablespoon of shredded coconut, 1 tablespoon of seeds, and 1 tablespoon of nuts. Garnish with lime zest (if using) and serve immediately.

INGREDIENT TIP: Macadamia nuts are an excellent source of quality fats, and their unique flavor pairs nicely with the coconut, but they can be pricey. Feel free to substitute another nut you may have on hand. Other "sweeter" nuts, such as pistachio, cashew, or pecan, would work well.

Per Serving: Calories: 408; Total Fat: 33g; Total Carbs: 17g; Net Carbs: 9g; Fiber: 8g; Protein: 16g; Sodium: 56mg; **Macros:** Fat: 73%, Carbs: 11%, Protein: 16%

CHERRY-COCONUT PANCAKES

Serves 3 | Prep Time: 5 minutes | Cook Time: 25 minutes | Gluten-Free, Vegetarian

This version of keto pancakes is grain-free, using a combination of almond meal and coconut flour for taste and texture. Almond meal is coarser and higher in fat and fiber than more refined almond flour, so it's worth seeking out. The powerful antioxidants in dark cherries help reduce inflammation and joint pain, so they are a healthy and delicious fruit to include in your diet. You can substitute a dark berry, such as raspberry or blackberry, if you have those on hand.

- 1 cup fresh or frozen dark cherries, thawed and coarsely chopped
- 1 tablespoon water or lemon juice
- 1 teaspoon vanilla extract, divided
- 2 to 4 teaspoons monk fruit extract or powdered sugar-free sweetener (optional)
- ½ cup almond meal
- ½ cup coconut flour
- ¼ cup ground flaxseed
- 1 teaspoon baking powder
- ½ teaspoon ground cinnamon
- ½ cup heavy whipping cream or full-fat canned coconut milk
- 1 large egg
- 2 tablespoons coconut oil, divided

1. In a small saucepan, heat the cherries, water, and ½ teaspoon of vanilla over medium-high heat for 5 to 6 minutes, until bubbly, adding more water if the mixture is too thick. Stir in the sweetener (if using). Using a fork, mash the cherries and whisk until the mixture is smooth. Remove from the heat and set aside.

2. In a large bowl, combine the almond meal, coconut flour, flaxseed, baking powder, and cinnamon and whisk to combine.

3. Add the cream, egg, 1 tablespoon of coconut oil, the remaining ½ teaspoon of vanilla, and a quarter of the cherry syrup mixture, whisking to combine well.

4. In large nonstick skillet, heat the remaining 1 tablespoon of coconut oil over medium-low heat. Using about 2 tablespoons of batter for each, form three pancakes. Cook for 4 to 5 minutes, until bubbles begin to form, then flip. Cook for 2 to 3 minutes on the second side, until the pancakes are golden brown. Repeat this process with the remaining batter. You should get six large pancakes. Serve warm drizzled with the remaining cherry syrup.

VARIATION TIP: Serve leftover pancakes with a smear of almond butter or sunflower seed butter for a delicious high-fat snack option. These pancakes freeze well.

Per Serving: Calories: 511; Total Fat: 41g; Total Carbs: 27g; Net Carbs: 14g; Fiber: 13g; Protein: 12g; Sodium: 236mg; **Macros:** Fat: 72%, Carbs: 19%, Protein: 9%

PUMPKIN PIE YOGURT BOWL

Serves 1 | Prep Time: 10 minutes | Egg-Free, Gluten-Free, Vegetarian

High in antioxidants, vitamin A, and fiber, pureed pumpkin is delicious and nutritious. As a starchy vegetable, pumpkin must be eaten in moderation on a ketogenic diet, but the addition of rich cream, pecans, and intense spice allows a little to go a long way. The bonus of anti-inflammatory properties from the cloves and cinnamon in pumpkin pie spice makes this a great option year-round.

1 tablespoon heavy whipping cream
½ cup plain whole milk Greek yogurt
1 tablespoon unsweetened pumpkin puree
1 teaspoon pumpkin pie spice (no sugar added)
1 to 2 teaspoons monk fruit extract or sugar-free sweetener (optional)
½ teaspoon vanilla extract
2 tablespoons coarsely chopped pecans

1. In a small bowl, using an immersion blender or whisk, whisk the cream for 2 to 3 minutes, until thick and doubled in volume. Set aside.

2. In a medium bowl, mix together the yogurt, pumpkin, pumpkin pie spice, sweetener (if using), and vanilla.

3. Top the yogurt mixture with the pecans and whipped cream and serve.

Per Serving: Calories: 266; Total Fat: 20g; Total Carbs: 9g; Net Carbs: 7g; Fiber: 2g; Protein: 13g; Sodium: 52mg;
Macros: Fat: 68%, Carbs: 12%, Protein: 20%

TOFU AND VEGGIE SCRAMBLE

Serves 2 | Prep Time: 10 minutes | Cook Time: 10 minutes | Dairy-Free, Egg-Free, Gluten-Free, Vegetarian

Variations of eggs are a common breakfast staple for ketogenic dieters, but every now and then you need to mix it up! Using tofu in place of eggs lends some variety and provides a vegan option for those needing a break from eggs. The anti-inflammatory super spice, turmeric, has a strong flavor and sometimes takes getting used to. Feel free to halve the quantity here until you are familiar with its flavor, which tends to be bitter in large quantities.

8 ounces firm tofu
¼ cup coconut oil, divided
2 tablespoons minced red onion
¼ red bell pepper, finely chopped
½ teaspoon ground turmeric
½ teaspoon salt
¼ teaspoon freshy ground black pepper
¼ teaspoon garlic powder
¼ cup chopped fresh cilantro or mint

1. Cut the block of tofu lengthwise into four pieces. Lay them flat on a stack of paper towels and drain for 5 minutes, pressing down with additional dry paper towels to release water.

2. Cut the drained tofu into chunks and place them in a large bowl. Using a fork, crumble the tofu into bite-size pieces.

3. In a medium skillet, heat 2 tablespoons of coconut oil over medium heat. Add the onion and bell pepper and sauté for 2 to 3 minutes, or until they are soft. Add the turmeric, salt, pepper, and garlic powder and sauté for 1 minute, or until fragrant. Add the remaining 2 tablespoons of coconut oil and stir to form a paste.

4. Add the crumbled tofu, increase the heat to medium high, and sauté for 3 to 4 minutes, until the tofu is slightly crispy.

5. Remove from the heat and stir in the cilantro. Serve warm.

Per Serving: Calories: 418; Total Fat: 37g; Total Carbs: 6g; Net Carbs: 3g; Fiber: 3g; Protein: 20g; Sodium: 608mg; **Macros:** Fat: 80%, Carbs: 1%, Protein: 19%

AVOCADO-MATCHA SMOOTHIE

Serves 1 | Prep Time: 5 minutes | Dairy-Free, Egg-Free, Gluten-Free

This rich and satiating green smoothie is full of antioxidant power from matcha, a green tea powder, and gut- and skin-health-boosting properties from the collagen protein. Feel free to use another no-carb protein powder of your choice.

- ¼ cup full-fat canned coconut milk, divided
- 1½ teaspoons matcha green tea powder
- 1 very ripe avocado, pitted and peeled
- 1 cup unsweetened almond milk
- 1 scoop unflavored collagen protein powder
- ½ teaspoon vanilla extract
- 1 to 2 teaspoons monk fruit extract or sugar-free sweetener

1. In a small microwave-safe bowl, heat 2 tablespoons of coconut milk in a small container in the microwave for 30 seconds.

2. Whisk the matcha into the hot milk until it's smooth.

3. In a blender or large wide-mouth jar (if using an immersion blender), combine the avocado, matcha mixture, the remaining 2 tablespoons of coconut milk, the almond milk, collagen powder, vanilla, and sweetener. Blend until smooth and creamy, adding more almond milk to achieve your desired consistency. Serve.

Per Serving: Calories: 424; Total Fat: 34g; Total Carbs: 17g; Net Carbs: 6g; Fiber: 11g; Protein: 17g; Sodium: 225mg;
Macros: Fat: 72%, Carbs: 12%, Protein: 16%

BLUEBERRY SMOOTHIE WITH LEMON AND GINGER

Serves 1 | Prep Time: 5 minutes | Dairy-Free, Egg-Free, Gluten-Free, Vegetarian

The lemon-ginger flavor in this refreshing smoothie complements the blueberry so nicely you don't want to dilute it with any other strong flavors. To keep fat content high, I add coconut oil, but be sure to use a filtered version in this recipe to cut down on the strong coconut flavor. You can substitute avocado or MCT oil if preferred.

1 cup unsweetened almond milk, plus more as needed
¼ cup frozen blueberries
2 tablespoons coconut oil
1 to 2 teaspoons monk fruit extract or sugar-free sweetener (optional)
½ teaspoon vanilla extract
½ teaspoon ground ginger, or 1 tablespoon minced fresh ginger
Grated zest of 1 lemon

In a blender or large wide-mouth jar (if using an immersion blender), combine the almond milk, blueberries, coconut oil, sweetener (if using), vanilla, ginger, and lemon zest. Blend until smooth and creamy, adding more almond milk to achieve your desired consistency. Serve.

Per Serving: Calories: 319; Total Fat: 30g; Total Carbs: 10g; Net Carbs: 8g; Fiber: 2g; Protein: 2g; Sodium: 172mg;
Macros: Fat: 85%, Carbs: 12%, Protein: 3%

ALMOND BUTTER AND CACAO NIB SMOOTHIE

Serves 1 | Prep Time: 5 minutes | Egg-Free, Gluten-Free, Vegetarian

Full of antioxidants, micronutrients, and fiber, cacao nibs are made from crushed cocoa beans and add wonderful flavor and crunch to this rich smoothie. Feel free to substitute canned coconut milk for the cream to make a dairy-free version.

- 1 cup unsweetened almond milk, plus more as needed
- ¼ cup heavy whipping cream
- 2 tablespoons unsweetened almond butter
- 1 tablespoon unsweetened cocoa powder
- 1 tablespoon cacao nibs, plus more for serving
- 1 to 2 teaspoons monk fruit extract or sugar-free sweetener (optional)
- ½ teaspoon almond extract (optional)
- ½ teaspoon cinnamon

In a blender or large wide-mouth jar (if using an immersion blender), combine the almond milk, cream, almond butter, cocoa powder, cacao nibs, sweetener (if using), almond extract (if using), and cinnamon. Blend until smooth and creamy, adding more almond milk to achieve your desired consistency. Serve garnished with additional cacao nibs.

Per Serving: Calories: 506; Total Fat: 47g; Total Carbs: 16g; Net Carbs: 7g; Fiber: 9g; Protein: 11g; Sodium: 190mg; **Macros:** Fat: 84%, Carbs: 7%, Protein: 9%

CHAFFLE AND LOX

Serves 4 | Prep Time: 5 minutes | Cook Time: 10 minutes | Gluten-Free

While the "chaffle," a variation of a waffle made with egg and cheese, is low in carbohydrates, it is not keto-friendly on its own due to its high ratio of protein to fat. This recipe uses a chaffle as the base, with the addition of almond flour to make it more like bread, for a delicious and rich variation of bagels and lox. Enjoy!

2 large eggs
1 cup freshly shredded mozzarella cheese
¼ cup almond flour
1 teaspoon everything bagel seasoning
½ teaspoon baking powder
5 tablespoons extra-virgin olive oil, divided
4 ounces goat cheese
4 ounces smoked salmon
4 thin slices red onion
8 thin slices cucumber
1 tablespoon chopped capers

1. Heat a waffle maker on medium heat.

2. In a medium bowl, whisk together the eggs, cheese, almond flour, everything seasoning, baking powder, and 1 tablespoon of olive oil until smooth.

3. When the waffle maker is hot, pour in half the batter and cook for 3 to 4 minutes, or until the waffle is golden brown. Repeat with the remaining half of the batter.

4. Spread 1 ounce of goat cheese over each waffle half and top with 1 ounce of smoked salmon, 1 slice of red onion, 2 slices of cucumber, and chopped capers. Drizzle each with 1 tablespoon of olive oil and serve immediately.

VARIATION TIP: This is also delicious topped with a sliced avocado and a drizzle of olive oil and seasoning to round out the macros and make a complete meal.

Per Serving: Calories: 466; Total Fat: 40g; Total Carbs: 4g; Net Carbs: 3g; Fiber: 1g; Protein: 22g; Sodium: 733mg; **Macros:** Fat: 77%, Carbs 4%, Protein: 19%

Moroccan-Spiced Cauliflower Salad, page 55

CHAPTER FOUR

Soups and Salads

LEMONY CHICKEN SALAD WITH BLUEBERRIES AND FENNEL

Serves 4 | Prep Time: 5 minutes | Dairy-Free, Gluten-Free

With its strong anise, or black licorice flavor, fennel is a root vegetable in the carrot family, common in many Mediterranean dishes. Here I used fennel seed for a more convenient way to impart that unique flavor. If you have fresh fennel bulb on hand, feel free to substitute chopped fresh fennel for the celery and fennel seed for a true treat.

- ½ cup Anti-Inflammatory Mayo (page 148)
- ¼ cup extra-virgin olive oil
- Grated zest and juice of 1 lemon
- 1 teaspoon fennel seed, slightly crushed
- ½ teaspoon salt
- ¼ teaspoon freshly ground black pepper
- 2 cups shredded cooked chicken
- 2 celery stalks, finely chopped
- ½ cup fresh or frozen blueberries, halved
- ½ cup slivered almonds

1. In a medium bowl, combine the mayo, olive oil, lemon zest and juice, fennel, salt, and pepper and whisk well to combine.

2. Add the chicken, celery, blueberries, and almonds and stir to coat. Serve.

INGREDIENT TIP: You can double this recipe to have on hand for quick, easy lunches throughout the week, but be sure to omit the slivered almonds until just before serving to prevent them from getting soggy in the refrigerator.

Per Serving: Calories: 564; Total Fat: 51g; Total Carbs: 8g; Net Carbs: 5g; Fiber: 3g; Protein: 23g; Sodium: 505mg; **Macros:** Fat: 81%, Carbs: 3%, Protein: 16%

CHILLED AVOCADO-CILANTRO SOUP

Serves 4 | Prep Time: 10 minutes | Egg-Free, Gluten-Free, Nut-Free, Vegetarian

This creamy and flavorful cold soup is a much more satiating take on gazpacho, the chilled tomato soup common in Spain. Protein from the yogurt makes this a complete meal. Store leftover soup in an airtight container in the refrigerator to prevent browning.

- 2 ripe avocados, pitted and peeled
- ½ cup plain whole milk Greek yogurt
- ½ cup chopped fresh cilantro
- ¼ cup extra-virgin olive oil
- ¼ cup freshly squeezed lime juice (about 4 limes)
- 1 teaspoon salt
- 1 teaspoon onion powder
- ½ teaspoon freshly ground black pepper
- ½ teaspoon garlic powder
- ½ teaspoon ground turmeric
- ¼ cup roasted pumpkin seeds, for garnish (optional)

1. Place the avocados, yogurt, cilantro, olive oil, lime juice, salt, onion powder, pepper, garlic powder, and turmeric in a blender or a wide cylindrical container (if using an immersion blender). Blend until smooth and creamy.

2. Serve chilled, topped with the pumpkin seeds (if using).

Per Serving: Calories: 268; Total Fat: 25g; Total Carbs: 9g; Net Carbs: 4g; Fiber: 5g; Protein: 4g; Sodium: 609mg; **Macros:** Fat: 84%, Carbs: 10%, Protein: 6%

VEGAN CREAMY ASPARAGUS SOUP

Serves 4 | Prep Time: 5 minutes | Cook Time: 20 minutes | Dairy-Free, Egg-Free, Gluten-Free, Nut-Free, Vegetarian

I love the fresh spring flavors in this soup, and it is delicious served both warm and chilled. For a complete meal, serve a warm bowl topped with a fresh egg fried in olive oil or add leftover shredded chicken, Baked Spiced Tofu (page 71), or a few slices of quality prosciutto for protein.

- 6 tablespoons extra-virgin olive oil, divided
- 1 pound asparagus, trimmed and cut into 2-inch pieces
- ½ cup chopped scallions, green parts only
- 4 garlic cloves, minced
- 1 teaspoon salt
- ½ teaspoon red pepper flakes
- 2 cups vegetable or chicken stock
- 1 cup water
- ¼ cup tahini
- Grated zest and juice of 1 lemon
- 2 tablespoons roasted pumpkin seeds

1. In a medium saucepan, heat 2 tablespoons of olive oil over medium heat. Add the asparagus and sauté for 2 to 3 minutes, until it is just tender.
2. Add the scallions, garlic, salt, and red pepper flakes and sauté for 2 to 3 minutes, until fragrant.
3. Add the stock and water, increase the heat to high, and bring to a boil. Reduce the heat to low, cover, and simmer for 8 to 10 minutes, or until the vegetables are tender.
4. Remove from the heat and allow to cool slightly. Add the tahini, the remaining 4 tablespoons of olive oil, and the lemon zest and juice.
5. Using an immersion blender (or a stand blender, blending in batches), puree the mixture until smooth and creamy.
6. Serve warm garnished with the pumpkin seeds.

INGREDIENT TIP: Tahini, or ground sesame seed paste, gives this soup a creamy and unique flavor while keeping it dairy-free. You can substitute 4 ounces of goat cheese and an additional ¼ cup of stock in place of the tahini if you prefer an even richer texture and different flavor.

Per Serving: Calories: 329; Total Fat: 30g; Total Carbs: 12g; Net Carbs: 8g; Fiber: 4g; Protein: 7g; Sodium: 897mg; **Macros:** Fat: 82%, Carbs: 9%, Protein: 9%

GUACAMOLE SALAD

Serves 4 | Prep Time: 10 minutes | Dairy-Free, Egg-Free, Gluten-Free, Nut-Free, Vegetarian

This deliciously fresh and easy avocado salad is like a deconstructed bowl of guacamole and comes together in a flash. Add some grilled shrimp or crab meat for a complete meal reminiscent of fresh ceviche. This also complements a quick weeknight dinner of grilled chicken or steak wonderfully.

- 2 avocados, cut into 1-inch chunks
- 4 Roma tomatoes, quartered
- 1 green bell pepper, cut into 1-inch chunks
- ¼ red onion, thinly sliced
- ½ cup packed whole fresh cilantro leaves
- ¼ cup extra-virgin olive oil
- Juice of 2 limes
- 1 teaspoon salt
- ½ teaspoon freshly ground black pepper

1. In a medium bowl, combine the avocados, tomatoes, bell pepper, onion, and cilantro.

2. In a small bowl, whisk together the olive oil, lime juice, salt, and pepper and drizzle over the salad. Toss to coat well and serve immediately.

Per Serving: Calories: 258; Total Fat: 24g; Total Carbs: 12g; Net Carbs: 6g; Fiber: 6g; Protein: 2g; Sodium: 600mg;
Macros: Fat: 84%, Carbs: 13%, Protein: 3%

CURRIED TUNA SALAD WITH PEPITAS

Serves 2 | Prep Time: 10 minutes | Dairy-Free, Egg-Free, Gluten-Free, Nut-Free

Packed with heart-healthy and anti-inflammatory monounsaturated fatty acids from avocado and olive oil, as well as intense flavor from herbs and spices, this tuna salad is a great staple to keep on hand in the refrigerator for a quick meal or filling snack. Enjoy on its own, atop a bed of mixed greens, or in lettuce wraps, or make a sandwich with a Keto Sandwich Round (page 146).

1 ripe avocado, halved and pitted
Juice of 1 lime
1 tablespoon avocado or extra-virgin olive oil
1 teaspoon curry powder
½ teaspoon salt
1 (4-ounce) can olive oil–packed tuna
2 tablespoons chopped fresh cilantro
2 tablespoons roasted pumpkin seeds

1. Using a spoon, scoop the avocado flesh into a medium bowl and mash well with a fork.

2. Add the lime juice, avocado oil, curry powder, and salt and mix well. Add the tuna and its oil, cilantro, and pumpkin seeds and mix well with a fork.

3. Eat immediately or store covered in the refrigerator for up to three days.

Per Serving: Calories: 347; Total Fat: 26g; Total Carbs: 9g; Net Carbs: 3g; Fiber: 6g; Protein: 22g; Sodium: 854mg; **Macros:** Fat: 67%, Carbs: 8%, Protein: 25%

ROASTED RED PEPPER SOUP WITH BASIL AND GOAT CHEESE

Serves 4 | Prep Time: 5 minutes | Cook Time: 15 minutes | Egg-Free, Gluten-Free, Nut-Free, Vegetarian

Sparking childhood memories of grilled cheese sandwiches and creamy tomato soup, this keto-friendly version is one of my favorite rainy-day treats. Using jarred roasted red peppers makes this a quick and easy weekday meal, but feel free to roast your own peppers for a deeper flavor if you have the time. Pair with a Keto Sandwich Round (page 146) for a true comfort meal.

- 6 tablespoons extra-virgin olive oil, divided
- ½ small onion, coarsely chopped
- 1 (16-ounce) jar roasted red peppers, drained and coarsely chopped
- 2 garlic cloves, minced
- 1 teaspoon salt
- ½ teaspoon freshly ground black pepper
- 3 cups vegetable or chicken stock
- 1 cup water
- 4 ounces goat cheese
- ½ cup chopped fresh basil
- 2 tablespoons red wine vinegar

1. In a medium saucepan, heat 2 tablespoons of olive oil over medium heat. Add the onion and sauté for 3 to 4 minutes, or until the onion has softened.
2. Add the red peppers, garlic, salt, and pepper and sauté for 2 to 3 minutes, or until fragrant.
3. Add the stock and water, increase the heat to high, and bring to a boil. Reduce the heat to low, cover, and simmer for 4 to 5 minutes to allow flavors to blend.
4. Remove from the heat and mix in the goat cheese, basil, the remaining 4 tablespoons of olive oil, and the vinegar.
5. Using an immersion blender (or a stand blender, blending in batches), puree the mixture until smooth and creamy.
6. Serve warm, garnished with additional basil.

Per Serving: Calories: 331; Total Fat: 29g; Total Carbs: 10g; Net Carbs: 8g; Fiber: 2g; Protein: 7g; Sodium: 1364mg; **Macros:** Fat: 79%, Carbs: 13%, Protein: 8%

CREAM OF MUSHROOM AND FENNEL SOUP

Serves 4 | Prep Time: 10 minutes | Cook Time: 25 minutes | Egg-Free, Gluten-Free, Nut-Free, Vegetarian

Most canned mushroom soups are not only full of inflammatory preservatives but also typically higher in carbohydrates and lacking in flavor. Fresh fennel and mushrooms (I prefer shiitake) give this rich version a starring role in any meal, rather than serve as a filler for grandma's casserole. You'll never reach for the store-bought version again!

2 tablespoons unsalted butter
1 cup sliced fennel bulb
8 ounces mushrooms, sliced and divided
2 garlic cloves, minced
2 tablespoons chopped fresh thyme or rosemary
1 teaspoon salt
½ teaspoon freshly ground black pepper
2 cups vegetable or beef stock
½ cup heavy whipping cream
2 tablespoons extra-virgin olive oil

1. In a medium saucepan, heat the butter over medium heat. Add the fennel and sauté for 5 to 6 minutes, or until the fennel is tender and slightly browned.

2. Add 6 ounces of mushrooms, garlic, thyme, salt, and pepper and sauté for 3 to 4 minutes, until the mushrooms are just soft.

3. Add the stock, increase the heat to high, and bring to a boil. Reduce the heat to low, cover and simmer for about 5 minutes, until the vegetables are very tender.

4. Remove from the heat and allow to cool slightly. Add the cream and olive oil and using an immersion blender (or a stand blender, blending in batches), puree the mixture until smooth and creamy.

5. Coarsely chop the remaining 2 ounces of mushrooms. If using a blender, return the creamed soup to the saucepan and heat over low. Add the mushrooms and cook, stirring constantly, for 3 to 4 minutes, or until the mushrooms are tender. Serve warm.

INGREDIENT TIP: Fresh fennel bulb gives this soup great flavor, and it's worth seeking out. However, you can substitute sliced onion for the fresh fennel and add 2 teaspoons of fennel seed for flavor.

Per Serving: Calories: 247; Total Fat: 24g; Total Carbs: 7g; Net Carbs: 5g; Fiber: 2g; Protein: 4g; Sodium: 875mg; **Macros:** Fat: 87%, Carbs: 7%, Protein: 6%

MOROCCAN-SPICED CAULIFLOWER SALAD

Serves 4 | Prep Time: 5 minutes | Cook Time: 25 minutes, plus 15 minutes to cool | Dairy-Free, Egg-Free, Gluten-Free, Vegetarian

Cauliflower tends to be a common staple on many ketogenic diets due its versatility as a stand-in for many higher-carb vegetables and grains. The intense flavors in this salad bring new life to this much-used vegetable.

- 4 cups fresh or frozen cauliflower florets
- 2 tablespoons coconut oil, melted
- 1 teaspoon salt, divided
- ¼ cup extra-virgin olive oil
- Grated zest and juice of 1 lemon
- 1 teaspoon chili powder
- 1 teaspoon ground cinnamon
- 1 teaspoon garlic powder
- ½ teaspoon ground turmeric
- ½ teaspoon ground ginger
- 2 celery stalks, thinly sliced
- ½ cup finely sliced fresh mint
- ¼ cup finely sliced red onion
- ¼ cup shelled pistachios

1. If using frozen cauliflower, thaw to room temperature in a colander, draining off any excess water. Cut larger florets into bite-size pieces.
2. Preheat the oven to 450°F and line a baking sheet with aluminum foil.
3. In a medium bowl, toss the cauliflower with coconut oil and ½ teaspoon of salt. Arrange the cauliflower in a single layer on the prepared baking sheet, reserving the seasoned bowl.
4. Roast the cauliflower for 20 to 25 minutes, until it is lightly browned and crispy.
5. While the cauliflower roasts, in the reserved bowl, whisk together the olive oil, lemon zest and juice, the remaining ½ teaspoon of salt, the chili powder, cinnamon, garlic powder, turmeric, and ginger. Stir in the celery, mint, and onion.
6. When the cauliflower is done roasting, remove from the oven and allow to cool for 10 to 15 minutes.
7. Toss the warm (but not too hot) cauliflower with the dressing until well combined. Add the pistachios and toss to incorporate. Serve warm or chilled.

MAKE AHEAD: You can serve this warm or at room temperature, but chilled leftovers taste even better the next day.

Per Serving: Calories: 262; Total Fat: 24g; Total Carbs: 11g; Net Carbs: 7g; Fiber: 4g; Protein: 4g; Sodium: 651mg; **Macros:** Fat: 82%, Carbs: 12%, Protein: 6%

CREAMY RICED CAULIFLOWER SALAD

Serves 4 | Prep Time: 10 minutes, plus 30 minutes to chill | Gluten-Free, Nut-Free, Vegetarian

This is my spin on a Greek-inspired orzo (rice-shaped pasta) salad my dad used to make for every barbecue or potluck. Even as a kid, I had a strong appreciation for the unique flavors of dill, feta, lemon, and olive. This low-carb version full of healthy fats is a new use for ubiquitous cauliflower rice.

- 4 ounces crumbled sheep's milk feta cheese
- ½ cup Anti-Inflammatory Mayo (page 148)
- Grated zest and juice of 1 lemon
- 2 tablespoons minced red onion
- 1½ teaspoons dried dill
- ½ teaspoon salt
- 1 teaspoon red pepper flakes, or to taste
- 3 cups fresh riced cauliflower (not frozen)
- ½ cup coarsely chopped pitted Kalamata olives

1. In a medium bowl, combine the feta, mayo, lemon zest and juice, onion, dill, salt, and red pepper flakes. Whisk well with a fork until smooth and creamy.

2. Add the cauliflower and olives and mix well to combine.

3. Refrigerate for at least 30 minutes before serving.

VARIATION TIP: The creamy feta dressing and mix-ins would also be delicious served with shredded cabbage for a unique spin on coleslaw.

Per Serving: Calories: 370; Total Fat: 37g; Total Carbs: 6g; Net Carbs: 4g; Fiber: 2g; Protein: 7g; Sodium: 1048mg; **Macros:** Fat: 90%, Carbs: 2%, Protein: 8%

LOADED MISO SOUP WITH TOFU AND EGG

Serves 4 | Prep Time: 10 minutes | Cook Time: 20 minutes | Dairy-Free, Gluten-Free, Nut-Free, Vegetarian

Miso is a paste made from fermented soybeans, but unlike soy sauce, without the addition of grains. Common in Asian cuisine, miso is usually stocked in the refrigerated produce or dairy (although it contains no dairy!) sections of grocery stores. This hearty and satisfying version of miso soup is loaded with anti-inflammatory vegetables, spices, and seaweed.

- 3 cups water
- 3 cups vegetable broth
- 3 tablespoons white miso paste
- 1 (2-inch) piece fresh ginger, peeled and minced
- 4 baby bok choy, trimmed and quartered
- 2 cups thinly sliced shiitake mushrooms
- 2 garlic cloves, very thinly sliced
- 1 (14-ounce) package firm tofu, drained and cut into bite-size cubes
- 2 cups spiralized or thinly sliced zucchini
- 2 large hard-boiled eggs, peeled and quartered
- 2 nori seaweed sheets, cut into very thin 2-inch strips
- ¼ cup avocado or extra-virgin olive oil
- 2 teaspoons toasted sesame oil

1. In a large saucepan, bring the water and vegetable broth to a boil over high heat. Reduce the heat to low, whisk in the miso paste and ginger, cover and simmer for 2 minutes.

2. Add the bok choy, mushrooms, and garlic. Simmer, covered, for 5 minutes, or until the vegetables are tender. Remove from the heat and stir in the tofu and zucchini.

3. Divide the mixture between bowls. Add 2 egg quarters and the seaweed strips to each bowl. Drizzle 1 tablespoon of avocado oil and ½ teaspoon of sesame oil over each bowl. Serve warm.

Per Serving: Calories: 378; Total Fat: 29g; Total Carbs: 14g; Net Carbs: 8g; Fiber: 6g; Protein: 17g; Sodium: 912mg; **Macros:** Fat: 69%, Carbs: 13%, Protein: 18%

WEEKDAY OMEGA-3 SALAD

Serves 2 | Prep Time: 10 minutes | Dairy-Free, Gluten-Free, Nut-Free

This salad is my go-to for a quick and easy lunch. Loaded with heart-healthy and anti-inflammatory omega-3 fatty acids, it is a fresh and satiating way to fuel your busy day! I am always sure to have a few cans of quality tuna or mackerel packed in olive oil in the pantry for a last-minute meal, but feel free to substitute fresh fish for the canned.

- 6 cups baby arugula or spinach
- 1 (4-ounce) can olive oil–packed tuna, mackerel, or salmon
- ¼ cup minced fresh parsley
- 10 green or black olives, pitted and halved
- 2 tablespoons minced scallions, white and green parts, or red onion
- 1 avocado, thinly sliced
- ¼ cup roasted pumpkin or sunflower seeds
- 6 tablespoons Basic Vinaigrette (page 147) or Caesar Dressing (page 144)

1. Divide the greens between bowls.

2. In a small bowl, combine the tuna and its oil with the parsley, olives, and scallions. Divide the fish mixture evenly on top of the greens.

3. Divide the avocado slices and pumpkin seeds between the bowls. Drizzle each with the dressing and toss to coat.

INGREDIENT TIP: I recommend always having Basic Vinaigrette or Caesar Dressing prepared in the refrigerator, but you can make an easy substitution by simply drizzling 2 tablespoons of extra-virgin olive oil and the juice of 1 lemon over the salad and tossing to coat.

Per Serving: Calories: 716; Total Fat: 61g; Total Carbs: 16g; Net Carbs: 5g; Fiber: 11g; Protein: 31g; Sodium: 1021mg; **Macros:** Fat: 77%, Carbs: 6%, Protein: 17%

CLASSIC COLESLAW

Serves 4 | Prep Time: 15 minutes, plus 30 minutes to chill | Dairy-Free, Gluten-Free, Nut-Free, Vegetarian

While they may seem like a healthy option, store-bought prepared coleslaws are full of added sugars, which are inflammatory and will prevent ketosis. This homemade alternative combines a variety of cruciferous vegetables, omega-3 fatty acids, and anti-inflammatory herbs and spices for flavor and health. I like to use the more tender Napa or savoy cabbages for the green cabbage in this recipe.

½ cup Anti-Inflammatory Mayo (page 148)
1 tablespoon avocado or extra-virgin olive oil
1 tablespoon Dijon mustard
1 tablespoon freshly squeezed lemon juice or apple cider vinegar
1 teaspoon salt
½ teaspoon ground turmeric
½ teaspoon freshly ground black pepper
3 cups shredded green cabbage
1 cup shredded red cabbage
1 cup coarsely chopped baby spinach leaves
½ cup chopped fresh cilantro, basil, or parsley
¼ small red onion, thinly sliced
¼ cup roasted pumpkin seeds or slivered almonds

1. In a small bowl, whisk together the mayo, avocado oil, mustard, lemon juice, salt, turmeric, and pepper. Set aside.

2. In a large bowl, combine the green and red cabbages, spinach, cilantro, and red onion. Add the dressing and toss to coat well. Refrigerate for at least 30 minutes to allow flavors to develop.

3. Serve chilled, topped with the pumpkin seeds.

VARIATION TIP: You can add 1 to 2 tablespoons of monk fruit extract or sugar-free sweetener of your choice if you find turmeric to be bitter.

Per Serving: Calories: 349; Total Fat: 35g; Total Carbs: 7g; Net Carbs: 4g; Fiber: 3g; Protein: 4g; Sodium: 856mg; **Macros:** Fat: 90%, Carbs: 5%, Protein: 5%

WEEKNIGHT GREEK SALAD

Serves 4 | Prep Time: 5 minutes | Egg-Free, Gluten-Free, Nut-Free, Vegetarian

Simple and deliciously nutritious, this traditional Greek salad includes marinated veggies for extra detoxifying properties and flavor. Traditional Greek feta is made with sheep's milk, not cow's, and tastes far superior to the more processed American versions. Top this salad with grilled chicken or fish, sliced hard-boiled egg, or Baked Spiced Tofu (page 71) for a complete meal.

- 8 cups coarsely chopped romaine lettuce
- 4 ounces crumbled sheep's milk feta cheese
- ½ cup Marinated Antipasto Veggies (page 133) or store-bought marinated artichoke hearts
- 20 Kalamata olives, pitted
- 2 tablespoons chopped fresh oregano or rosemary, or 2 teaspoons dried oregano
- ¼ cup extra-virgin olive oil
- Juice of 1 lemon
- ½ teaspoon freshly ground black pepper

In a large bowl, combine the lettuce, feta, antipasto veggies, olives, and oregano. Drizzle with the olive oil, then add the lemon juice and pepper. Toss to coat and serve immediately.

Per Serving: Calories: 300; Total Fat: 27g; Total Carbs: 10g; Net Carbs: 7g; Fiber: 3g; Protein: 6g; Sodium: 795mg; **Macros:** Fat: 81%, Carbs: 11%, Protein: 8%

ITALIAN GREEN BEAN SALAD

Serves 4 | Prep Time: 5 minutes | Cook Time: 5 minutes, plus 1 hour to chill | Dairy-Free, Egg-Free, Gluten-Free, Vegetarian

With anti-inflammatory fresh herbs and garlic, this easy side is full of healthy flavor. I prefer this served cold, and it is a wonderful addition to any backyard barbecue. Feel free to substitute asparagus for the green beans if it's in season.

¼ cup extra-virgin olive oil, divided
1 pound green beans, trimmed
2 tablespoons red wine vinegar
1 teaspoon salt
1 teaspoon red pepper flakes
2 garlic cloves, thinly sliced
½ cup slivered almonds
¼ cup thinly sliced fresh basil
2 tablespoons chopped fresh mint

1. In a large skillet, heat 2 tablespoons of olive oil over medium-high heat. Add the green beans and sauté for about 5 minutes, until they are just tender. Remove from the heat and transfer to a large serving bowl.

2. In a small bowl, whisk together the remaining 2 tablespoons of olive oil, the vinegar, salt, red pepper flakes, and garlic. Pour the dressing over the green beans and toss to coat well.

3. Add the almonds, basil, and mint and toss well. Serve warm or chill for at least 1 hour to serve cold.

Per Serving: Calories: 238; Total Fat: 21g; Total Carbs: 12g; Net Carbs: 7g; Fiber: 5g; Protein: 5g; Sodium: 598mg; **Macros:** Fat: 79%, Carbs: 13%, Protein: 8%

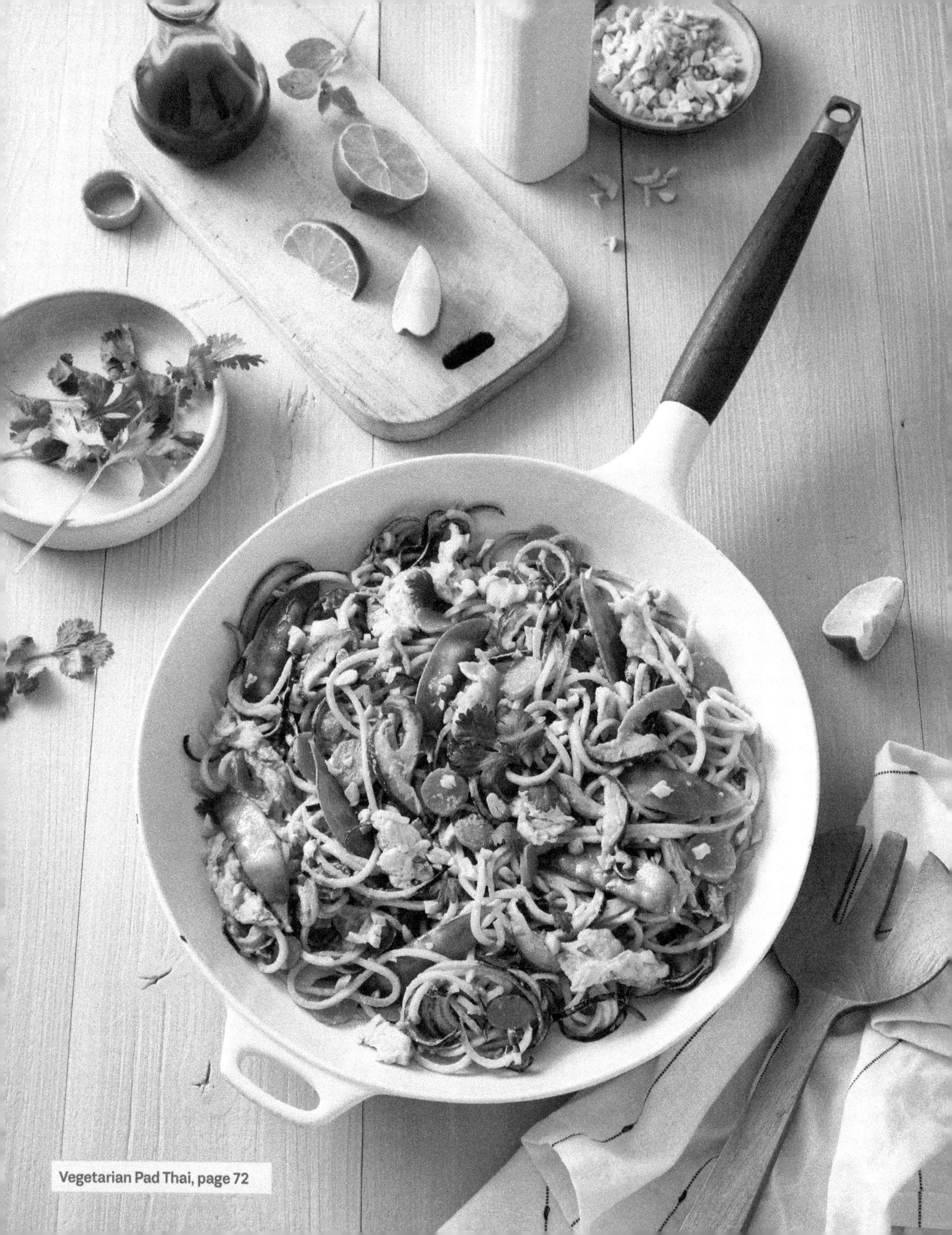

Vegetarian Pad Thai, page 72

CHAPTER FIVE

Vegetarian Dishes

CRISPY TOFU WITH MUSHROOMS AND BOK CHOY

Serves 4 | Prep Time: 10 minutes | Cook Time: 25 minutes | Dairy-Free, Egg-Free, Gluten-Free, Vegetarian

Asian mushrooms, such as shiitake, contain immune-protecting properties and powerful anti-inflammatory agents. They are far superior to mass-produced varieties such as cremini or portabella, and are worth spending a bit extra on. Red curry paste adds a rich flavor and can be found in the international aisle of most grocery stores, but you can use red pepper flakes in a pinch.

- 1 (14-ounce) package extra-firm tofu, drained
- ¼ cup tamari
- 2 tablespoons unsweetened almond or cashew butter
- 1 tablespoon rice vinegar
- 1 tablespoon sesame oil
- 1 teaspoon red curry paste or red pepper flakes
- ¼ cup coconut oil
- 1 (2-inch) piece fresh ginger, peeled and minced
- 4 baby bok choy, trimmed and quartered
- 4 ounces shiitake mushrooms, sliced
- 4 garlic cloves, thinly sliced

1. Preheat the oven to 400°F and line a baking sheet with parchment paper.

2. Cut the tofu into ½-inch cubes and arrange them at least ½ inch apart in a single layer on the prepared baking sheet. Bake on the middle rack of the oven for 15 to 20 minutes, or until the tofu is golden and crispy, being careful not to burn it. Remove from the oven.

3. While the tofu bakes, in a small bowl, whisk together the tamari, almond butter, rice vinegar, sesame oil, and red curry paste. Set aside.

4. In large skillet, heat the coconut oil over medium-high heat. Add the ginger and sauté for 2 to 3 minutes, until fragrant. Add the bok choy and mushrooms and sauté for 5 to 6 minutes, until they are just tender and wilted.

5. Add the garlic and sauté for 1 minute, or until fragrant. Pour the reserved tamari mixture over the vegetables, add the baked tofu, and stir to coat well. Reduce the heat to low, cover, and simmer for 3 to 4 minutes, or until the sauce is slightly thickened.

6. Uncover, toss to coat, and serve warm.

INGREDIENT TIP: This is delicious with a variety of vegetables such as green beans or broccoli. Adjust the sautéing time as needed.

Per Serving: Calories: 340; Total Fat: 27g; Total Carbs: 10g; Net Carbs: 6g; Fiber: 4g; Protein: 16g; Sodium: 1109mg; **Macros:** Fat: 71%, Carbs: 10%, Protein: 19%

LEMON-HERB BAKED FRITTATA

Serves 4 | Prep Time: 5 minutes | Cook Time: 40 minutes, plus 10 minutes to cool | Gluten-Free, Nut-Free, Vegetarian

Frittatas, baked egg dishes typically made with vegetables and cheese, are common in many European cuisines. They take on a variety of different flavors and textures, depending on the vegetables and herbs used. This version is heavier on the cheese for a creamy texture and is prepared exclusively in the oven, as opposed to the stovetop, for ease. It's delicious served at brunch or atop a salad for a light lunch.

- 6 tablespoons extra-virgin olive oil, divided
- 8 ounces sheep's milk feta cheese
- 2 tablespoons chopped fresh rosemary
- 1 tablespoon chopped fresh oregano
- 1 teaspoon garlic powder
- 1 teaspoon grated lemon zest
- ½ teaspoon freshly ground black pepper
- 4 large eggs
- ½ teaspoon baking powder

1. Preheat the oven to 350°F.
2. Pour 2 tablespoons of olive oil into an 8-inch square glass baking dish and swirl to coat the bottom.
3. In a medium bowl, crumble the feta using a fork. Add the rosemary, oregano, garlic powder, lemon zest, and pepper and mix well.
4. In a small bowl, whisk together the eggs and baking powder. Add the egg mixture and the remaining 4 tablespoons of olive oil to the feta mixture and whisk well to combine.
5. Pour the egg mixture into the prepared baking dish and bake for 35 to 40 minutes, until it is lightly browned and set. Remove from the oven and allow to cool for 10 minutes. Slice and serve.

Per Serving: Calories: 412; Total Fat: 38g; Total Carbs: 4g; Net Carbs: 4g; Fiber: <1g; Protein: 15g; Sodium: 770mg; **Macros:** Fat: 83%, Carbs: 2%, Protein: 15%

MUSHROOM AND WALNUT SLIDERS

Serves 4 | Prep Time: 10 minutes | Cook Time: 10 minutes | Gluten-Free, Vegetarian

The earthy flavor from mushrooms and sage combined with the richness of walnuts really makes for a savory and filling meat-alternative burger. Due to the high water content of mushrooms, the mixture will get soggy if it sits too long before cooking, so be sure to prep these only when you are ready to cook them right away. They are delicious on their own, crumbled over a salad, in a lettuce wrap, or inside a Keto Sandwich Round (page 146).

- 1 cup walnut pieces
- 1 (8-ounce) package sliced mushrooms (preferably shiitake)
- 1 bunch scallions, white and green parts, coarsely chopped (about ½ cup)
- 12 large fresh sage leaves
- 3 large garlic cloves, peeled
- 1 large egg
- 1½ teaspoons salt, divided
- 1 teaspoon freshly ground black pepper, divided
- ½ cup almond meal
- ¼ cup extra-virgin olive oil, divided
- 1 large avocado, mashed
- 2 ounces goat cheese, at room temperature

1. In the bowl of a food processor, pulse the walnuts until well chopped but not quite a fine meal. Transfer to a large bowl.

2. In the food processor, combine the mushrooms, scallions, sage, and garlic and process until they form a thick paste. Add the mushroom mixture to the walnuts in the bowl.

3. In a small bowl, whisk together the egg with 1 teaspoon of salt and ½ teaspoon of pepper. Add the egg mixture and almond meal to the mushroom mixture and mix with a fork until well combined.

4. Immediately form into eight patties, about 2 inches in diameter.

5. In a large nonstick skillet, heat 2 tablespoons of olive oil over medium-high heat. Fry the sliders for 4 minutes. Carefully flip each slider, using tongs if necessary to avoid crumbling. Cover the skillet, reduce the heat to medium-low, and cook for 4 to 5 minutes, until they are set.

6. While the sliders cook, combine the remaining 2 tablespoons of olive oil, the avocado, and goat cheese in a small bowl and whisk until smooth. Season with the remaining ½ teaspoon of salt and ½ teaspoon of pepper.

7. Serve the sliders topped with the avocado-goat cheese mixture.

MAKE AHEAD: These freeze well, so you can double or triple the recipe to have leftovers ready for a last-minute meal. Fully cook the burgers according to the recipe and cool completely. Wrap each slider individually in aluminum foil and store in a resealable bag in the freezer for up to three months. To reheat, place a frozen slider on a foil-lined baking sheet and bake at 375°F for 10 to 15 minutes, until heated through.

Per Serving: Calories: 545; Total Fat: 50g; Total Carbs: 17g; Net Carbs: 8g; Fiber: 9g; Protein: 14g; Sodium: 972mg; **Macros:** Fat: 83%, Carbs: 7%, Protein: 10%

RATATOUILLE WITH FENNEL

Serves 4 | Prep Time: 10 minutes | Cook Time: 30 minutes | Dairy-Free, Egg-Free, Gluten-Free, Nut-Free, Vegetarian

Ratatouille is a French stewed vegetable dish. Several variations exist, but eggplant, tomatoes, squash, and peppers—all keto-friendly nonstarchy vegetables—are commonly used. I have added fennel to this version, both for its wonderful anise flavor and its powerful antioxidant properties. It's worth seeking out, but if you can't find fresh fennel bulb, you can substitute fennel seed in its place.

½ cup extra-virgin olive oil
1 onion, thinly sliced
1 fennel bulb, white part only, bottom trimmed and thinly sliced
4 garlic cloves, minced
1 teaspoon smoked paprika
1 teaspoon salt
½ teaspoon freshly ground black pepper
½ teaspoon ground turmeric
1 eggplant, cut into 1-inch cubes
2 zucchini or yellow squash, cut into ½-inch thick rounds
4 Roma tomatoes, quartered
½ cup chopped parsley

1. In a large soup pot or Dutch oven, heat the olive oil over medium heat. Add the onion and fennel and sauté for 8 to 10 minutes, until they are softened and fragrant. Add the garlic, paprika, salt, pepper, and turmeric and sauté for 2 minutes, until fragrant.

2. Add the eggplant, zucchini, and tomatoes and sauté for 4 to 5 minutes, until the vegetables are just tender. Reduce the heat to low, cover, and cook, stirring occasionally, for 10 to 12 minutes, or until the vegetables are very tender.

3. Remove from the heat and stir in the parsley. Season to taste with salt and pepper and serve warm.

MAKE AHEAD: The vegetables can be prepped ahead of time and stored in separate bags in the refrigerator (one for the onions and fennel and another for the eggplant, zucchini, and tomatoes) for a quick weeknight vegetarian meal. Top each serving with a fried egg or Baked Spiced Tofu (page 71).

Per Serving: Calories: 340; Total Fat: 28g; Total Carbs: 23g; Net Carbs: 14g; Fiber: 9g; Protein: 5g; Sodium: 640mg; **Macros:** Fat: 74%, Carbs: 20%, Protein: 6%

SOUTHWESTERN STUFFED PEPPERS

Serves 4 | Prep Time: 5 minutes | Cook Time: 35 minutes | Egg-Free, Gluten-Free, Nut-Free, Vegetarian

Colorful bell peppers are high in antioxidants and a wonderful addition to any healthy diet, but they are a bit higher in carbohydrates and natural sugars, so those following a ketogenic approach to reduce inflammation need to limit quantities. This recipe uses only half of a pepper per serving to reap all of the nutrition benefit without disrupting macronutrient ratios.

2 large bell peppers, any color
1 (14-ounce) package extra-firm tofu, drained
1 teaspoon garlic powder
1 teaspoon salt
1 teaspoon chili powder
6 tablespoons extra-virgin olive oil, divided
4 ounces crumbled sheep's milk feta cheese (optional)
½ cup chopped fresh cilantro
¼ cup roasted pumpkin seeds

1. Preheat the oven to 400°F.
2. Halve each pepper lengthwise. Remove the stem, seeds, and membrane.
3. In a large bowl, place the tofu and, using a knife, crumble well. Add the garlic powder, salt, and chili powder and mix well to coat.
4. In a skillet, heat 2 tablespoons of olive oil over medium-high heat. Add the crumbled tofu and sauté, stirring constantly, for 5 to 6 minutes, until it is crispy and most of the water has evaporated. Remove from the heat and stir in the feta (if using), cilantro, and pumpkin seeds.
5. Divide the mixture evenly between the four pepper halves, packing down as needed.
6. Drizzle each pepper half with 1 tablespoon of olive oil and bake for 25 to 30 minutes, until the tops are golden and peppers are tender.

VARIATION TIP: You can use mini snack-size sweet peppers or jalapeños for a fun appetizer. To feed a crowd, use the full recipe for the tofu mixture. For a smaller batch, halve the tofu, spices, and oil.

Per Serving: Calories: 350; Total Fat: 29g; Total Carbs: 10g; Net Carbs: 6g; Fiber: 4g; Protein: 14g; Sodium: 621mg; **Macros:** Fat: 75%, Carbs: 9%, Protein: 16%

OMEGA-3 GRAIN-FREE BOWL

Serves 4 | Prep Time: 10 minutes | Cook Time: 5 minutes | Dairy-Free, Egg-Free, Gluten-Free, Vegetarian

Who doesn't love a one-bowl meal? So many bowls include grains as the main base, which definitely don't work on a ketogenic diet. This grain-free version is so tasty and satisfying, you won't miss the filler starchy grain!

- ½ cup coarsely chopped walnuts
- ¼ cup coarsely chopped pistachios
- ¼ cup raw pumpkin seeds or sunflower seeds
- 4 cups baby arugula or spinach leaves
- 2 cups riced cauliflower (not frozen)
- 1 large seedless cucumber, peeled and chopped
- 4 Roma tomatoes, seeded and chopped
- ½ cup chopped parsley or cilantro
- ¼ cup chopped red onion
- ¼ cup extra-virgin olive oil
- 2 tablespoons apple cider vinegar
- 1 teaspoon salt
- ¼ teaspoon freshly ground black pepper

1. In a large dry skillet, toast the walnuts, pistachios, and pumpkin seeds over medium-low heat for about 5 minutes, until the nuts and seeds are golden and fragrant. Remove from the skillet and set aside to cool.

2. In a large bowl, combine the arugula, cauliflower, cucumber, tomatoes, parsley, and onion.

3. In a small bowl, whisk together the olive oil, vinegar, salt, and pepper. Add the cooled nuts and seeds to the vegetable bowl, drizzle with the oil mixture, and toss to coat well.

4. Divide among bowls and serve chilled or at room temperature.

INGREDIENT TIP: Frozen cauliflower retains a lot of extra water from the freezing process and tends to be mushy when thawed and used raw, such as in this recipe. Try making your own fresh Perfect Riced Cauliflower (page 156) or buying prepared fresh riced cauliflower available in the produce section of most grocery stores.

Per Serving: Calories: 349; Total Fat: 30g; Total Carbs: 14g; Net Carbs: 8g; Fiber: 6g; Protein: 10g; Sodium: 620mg; **Macros:** Fat: 77%, Carbs: 12%, Protein: 11%

BAKED SPICED TOFU

Serves 4 | Prep Time: 5 minutes | Cook Time: 20 minutes, plus 24 hours to marinate | Dairy-Free, Egg-Free, Gluten-Free, Nut-Free, Vegetarian

I like to keep this on hand in the refrigerator to put atop a salad for a quick and easy meatless meal. Many people are turned off by tofu, believing it to be bland and boring, but the flavors in this dish only get more intense as it marinates. I recommend letting it sit in the refrigerator for at least 24 hours before enjoying, although it can be eaten immediately after preparing.

- 2 teaspoons ground cumin
- 2 teaspoons smoked paprika
- 1 teaspoon ground cinnamon
- 1 teaspoon garlic powder
- 1 teaspoon ground turmeric
- 1 teaspoon red pepper flakes
- 1 teaspoon salt
- 1 (14-ounce) package extra-firm tofu, drained
- ⅓ cup extra-virgin olive oil
- 2 tablespoons tahini or unsweetened almond butter

1. Preheat the oven to 400°F and line a baking sheet with parchment paper.
2. In a small bowl, combine the cumin, paprika, cinnamon, garlic powder, turmeric, red pepper flakes, and salt. Place half of the spice mixture in a large bowl, reserving the other half.
3. Cut the tofu block into four large rectangles and place on several layers of paper towels. Cover with additional paper towels and press down to release the water. Cut the rectangles into 1-inch cubes and transfer to the bowl with the spice mixture. Toss to coat well.
4. Arrange the tofu cubes ½ inch apart in a single layer on the prepared baking sheet, reserving the bowl. Bake the tofu for 15 to 20 minutes, until it is crispy and golden.
5. While the tofu bakes, add the olive oil and tahini to the reserved spice mixture and whisk until smooth.
6. In the large reserved bowl, combine the baked tofu with the oil-tahini mixture and toss well to coat. Allow to cool completely if not serving warm.
7. Transfer to a storage container, cover and allow to marinate 24 hours refrigerated.

Per Serving: Calories: 321; Total Fat: 28g; Total Carbs: 8g; Net Carbs: 5g; Fiber: 3g; Protein: 12g; Sodium: 608mg;
Macros: Fat: 79%, Carbs: 6%, Protein: 15%

VEGETARIAN PAD THAI

Serves 4 | Prep Time: 15 minutes | Cook Time: 25 minutes | Dairy-Free, Gluten-Free, Vegetarian

A take-out favorite, pad Thai doesn't have to disappear just because you are focusing on your health! This version uses tamari, a wheat-free fermented soybean sauce, and zucchini noodles in place of pasta. This recipe calls for a wide variety of vegetables for a complex dish, but feel free to substitute what you have on hand for convenience.

- 3 large zucchini, spiralized (about 6 cups)
- 4 large eggs
- ¼ cup, plus 2 tablespoons tamari, divided
- 3 tablespoons sesame oil, divided
- ¼ cup avocado oil, divided
- ½ cup unsweetened almond or cashew butter
- Grated zest and juice of 1 lime
- 4 celery stalks, thinly sliced
- 1 carrot, peeled and thinly sliced into rounds
- 4 ounces shiitake mushrooms, thinly sliced
- 1 cup snow peas, trimmed
- 1 (2-inch) piece fresh ginger, peeled and minced
- ½ cup chopped scallions, white and green parts
- 2 garlic cloves, minced

1. Place the zucchini in a large bowl.

2. In a small bowl, whisk together the eggs, 2 tablespoons of tamari, and 2 tablespoons of sesame oil.

3. In a large nonstick skillet, heat 2 tablespoons of avocado oil over medium-high heat. Add the egg mixture, reduce the heat to medium, and cook undisturbed for 2 to 3 minutes, until the eggs begin to set. Using a rubber spatula, scramble the eggs for 2 to 3 minutes, until cooked through. Transfer the eggs to a plate or bowl to keep warm, reserving the skillet.

4. In another small bowl, combine the almond butter, lime zest and juice, the remaining ¼ cup of tamari, and the remaining 1 tablespoon of sesame oil and whisk until smooth.

5. In the reserved skillet, heat the remaining 2 tablespoons of avocado oil over medium heat. Add the celery, carrot, mushrooms, snow peas, and ginger and sauté for 4 to 5 minutes, until the vegetables are just tender. Add the scallions and garlic and sauté for 2 to 3 minutes. Add the almond butter mixture, reduce the heat to low, and cook, stirring constantly, for 3 to 4 minutes, until heated through.

¼ cup chopped fresh cilantro
¼ cup chopped fresh mint
¼ cup chopped cashews
1 lime, quartered

6. Pour the vegetable and sauce mixture over the zucchini, add the cooked egg, cilantro, mint, and cashews and toss to coat well.

7. Serve warm garnished with the lime wedges.

COOKING TIP: Simply tossing the zucchini with the warm sauce (rather than cooking it) helps retain its bite so that it does not get mushy.

Per Serving: Calories: 625; Total Fat: 51g; Total Carbs: 27g; Net Carbs: 18g; Fiber: 9g; Protein: 22g; Sodium: 1642mg; **Macros:** Fat: 73%, Carbs: 13%, Protein: 14%

TURMERIC AND AVOCADO EGG SALAD

Serves 2 | Prep Time: 10 minutes | Cook Time: 12 minutes, plus 1 hour to chill | Dairy-Free, Gluten-Free, Nut-Free, Vegetarian

A healthy updated spin on a classic, this egg salad replaces much of the saturated fat with heart-healthy monounsaturated fats. The addition of turmeric helps reduce inflammation while adding a unique flavor. Be sure to use free-range eggs for the best quality fats. Serve on its own or as a sandwich using a Keto Sandwich Round (page 146).

4 large eggs
1 avocado, halved and pitted
2 tablespoons Anti-Inflammatory Mayo (page 148)
1 tablespoon chopped capers
1 tablespoon minced red onion
½ teaspoon ground turmeric
½ teaspoon salt
Grated zest and juice of 1 lime
¼ teaspoon freshly ground black pepper
¼ cup chopped fresh cilantro (optional)

1. In a medium saucepan, place the eggs and cover with room temperature water.

2. Set a timer for 12 minutes, place the saucepan over high heat, and bring the water to a boil. Reduce the heat to medium and gently boil the eggs until the 12 minutes are up.

3. Remove the eggs from the hot water and soak them in a small bowl of ice water for 3 to 4 minutes, until they are cool to the touch.

4. While the eggs cool, using a spoon, scoop the avocado flesh into a medium bowl. Mash well with a fork. Add the mayo, capers, onion, turmeric, salt, lime zest and juice, and pepper and stir until well blended. Add the cilantro (if using), and stir to incorporate well.

5. Once the eggs have cooled, peel them and chop well. Add the eggs to the avocado mixture and stir to combine. Allow to chill in the refrigerator for at least 1 hour before serving.

Per Serving: Calories: 328; Total Fat: 30g; Total Carbs: 10g; Net Carbs: 5g; Fiber: 5g; Protein: 8g; Sodium: 836mg;
Macros: Fat: 82%, Carbs: 8%, Protein: 10%

MUSHROOM FAJITA LETTUCE WRAPS

Serves 4 | Prep Time: 15 minutes | Cook Time: 15 minutes | Egg-Free, Gluten-Free, Nut-Free, Vegetarian

The bulk of the active time in this easy weeknight meal is in the chopping of the veggies and garnishes, so I recommend prepping this ahead of time if you want a meal that can come together in a flash. Loaded with monounsaturated anti-inflammatory fats from avocados and oil, this light meal is surprisingly satiating!

6 tablespoons avocado oil, divided
2 zucchini cut into ½-inch-thick half moons
8 ounces portabella or shiitake mushrooms, sliced
1 bell pepper, any color, sliced
½ red onion, thinly sliced
1 teaspoon chili powder
1 teaspoon garlic powder
½ teaspoon cumin
½ teaspoon salt
8 large romaine, Bibb, or red leaf lettuce leaves
4 ounces crumbled sheep's milk feta cheese
1 recipe Spiced Guacamole (page 152)
2 tablespoons roasted pumpkin seeds
½ cup chopped fresh cilantro
Lime wedges

1. In a large nonstick skillet, heat 2 tablespoons of avocado oil over medium-high heat. Add the zucchini, mushrooms, bell pepper, and onion and sauté for 2 to 3 minutes. Add the chili powder, garlic powder, cumin, and salt and sauté for 6 to 8 minutes, until the vegetables are very tender. Remove from the heat.

2. Serve the warm vegetables in the lettuce leaves topped with the feta, guacamole, pumpkin seeds, and a drizzle of the remaining avocado oil (½ tablespoon per fajita). Garnish with the cilantro and lime juice.

Per Serving: Calories: 511; Total Fat: 47g; Total Carbs: 20g; Net Carbs: 11g; Fiber: 9g; Protein: 10g; Sodium: 1253mg; **Macros:** Fat: 83%, Carbs: 9%, Protein: 8%

SPINACH-ARTICHOKE TORTA

Serves 4 | Prep Time: 10 minutes | Cook Time: 1 hour | Gluten-Free, Nut-Free, Vegetarian

This heartier version of classic restaurant fare uses goat cheese instead of the traditional cream cheese or mayo for a wonderful flavor. The extra protein from the eggs makes a complete meal. Serve this atop a mixed-greens salad for a light lunch or cut it into smaller squares and serve as an appetizer or snack.

¼ cup extra-virgin olive oil, divided
½ onion, finely chopped
1 (14.5-ounce) can artichokes, drained and coarsely chopped
8 ounces frozen spinach, thawed and drained well
4 garlic cloves, minced
8 ounces goat cheese
1 teaspoon salt
1 teaspoon red pepper flakes
1 teaspoon dried oregano
6 large eggs
¼ cup heavy whipping cream
½ teaspoon baking powder
½ teaspoon salt
¼ teaspoon freshly ground black pepper
¼ cup chopped fresh basil, or 2 teaspoons dried basil
½ cup freshly shredded Parmesan cheese (optional)

1. Preheat the oven to 375°F.

2. In a large nonstick skillet, heat 2 tablespoons of olive oil over medium heat. Add the onion and sauté for 4 to 5 minutes, until it's lightly golden and soft. Add the artichokes, spinach, and garlic and sauté for 3 to 4 minutes, until heated through and any excess water has evaporated.

3. Add the goat cheese, salt, red pepper flakes, and oregano, reduce the heat to medium low, and stirring constantly, cook for 3 to 4 minutes, until the cheese is creamy and the mixture is well combined. Remove from the heat and allow to cool slightly.

4. In large bowl, whisk together the eggs, cream, baking powder, salt, and pepper. Add the cooled goat cheese, vegetable mixture, and basil and whisk to combine well.

5. In an 8-inch-square glass baking dish, drizzle the remaining 2 tablespoons of olive oil and swirl to coat the bottom. Pour the egg and cheese mixture into the prepared dish. Top with the Parmesan (if using), and bake for 30 to 35 minutes, until set. Remove from the oven and allow to cool at least 10 minutes, then slice and serve.

Per Serving: Calories: 564; Total Fat: 44g; Total Carbs: 14g; Net Carbs: 10g; Fiber: 4g; Protein: 27g; Sodium: 1653mg; **Macros:** Fat: 70%, Carbs: 11%, Protein: 19%

TOFU TIKKA MASALA

Serves 4 | Prep Time: 10 minutes | Cook Time: 25 minutes | Dairy-Free, Egg-Free, Gluten-Free, Vegetarian

This high-fat, low-carb variation of the take-out favorite cuts the carbs without compromising the flavor. Garam masala is a spice blend common in Indian and Middle Eastern cuisine and combines many anti-inflammatory spices, including cumin, coriander, cardamom, pepper, cinnamon, cloves, and nutmeg. It can be found in most grocery stores in the spice aisle.

¼ cup coconut oil
2 tablespoons extra-virgin olive oil
½ onion, finely chopped
1 (2-inch) piece fresh ginger, peeled and minced
4 garlic cloves, minced
1½ tablespoons garam masala
1 teaspoon fennel seed
1 (13.5-ounce) can full-fat coconut milk
½ cup vegetable broth
2 tablespoons tomato paste
1 teaspoon salt
1 (14-ounce) package extra-firm tofu, drained and cut into 1-inch cubes
Grated zest and juice of 1 lime
Perfect Riced Cauliflower (page 156) or steamed spinach, for serving
½ cup chopped fresh cilantro

1. In a large saucepan or Dutch oven, heat the coconut and olive oils over medium heat. Add the onion and ginger and sauté for 4 to 5 minutes, until the onion is lightly browned and just soft. Add the garlic, garam masala, and fennel and sauté for 2 to 3 minutes, until a thick paste has formed.

2. Whisk in the coconut milk, broth, tomato paste, and salt and bring to a boil over high heat. Reduce the heat to low, add the tofu, and simmer, covered, for 10 to 15 minutes, or until the flavors have developed. Remove from the heat and stir in the lime zest and juice.

3. Serve warm over riced cauliflower or steamed spinach, garnished with the cilantro.

VARIATION TIP: For a crispier tofu, bake the cubed tofu prior to adding it to the sauce mixture, or use Baked Spiced Tofu (page 71) for an intensely flavorful and crispy addition.

Per Serving: Calories: 473; Total Fat: 42g; Total Carbs: 14g; Net Carbs: 11g; Fiber: 3g; Protein: 13g; Sodium: 684mg;
Macros: Fat: 80%, Carbs; 9%, Protein: 11%

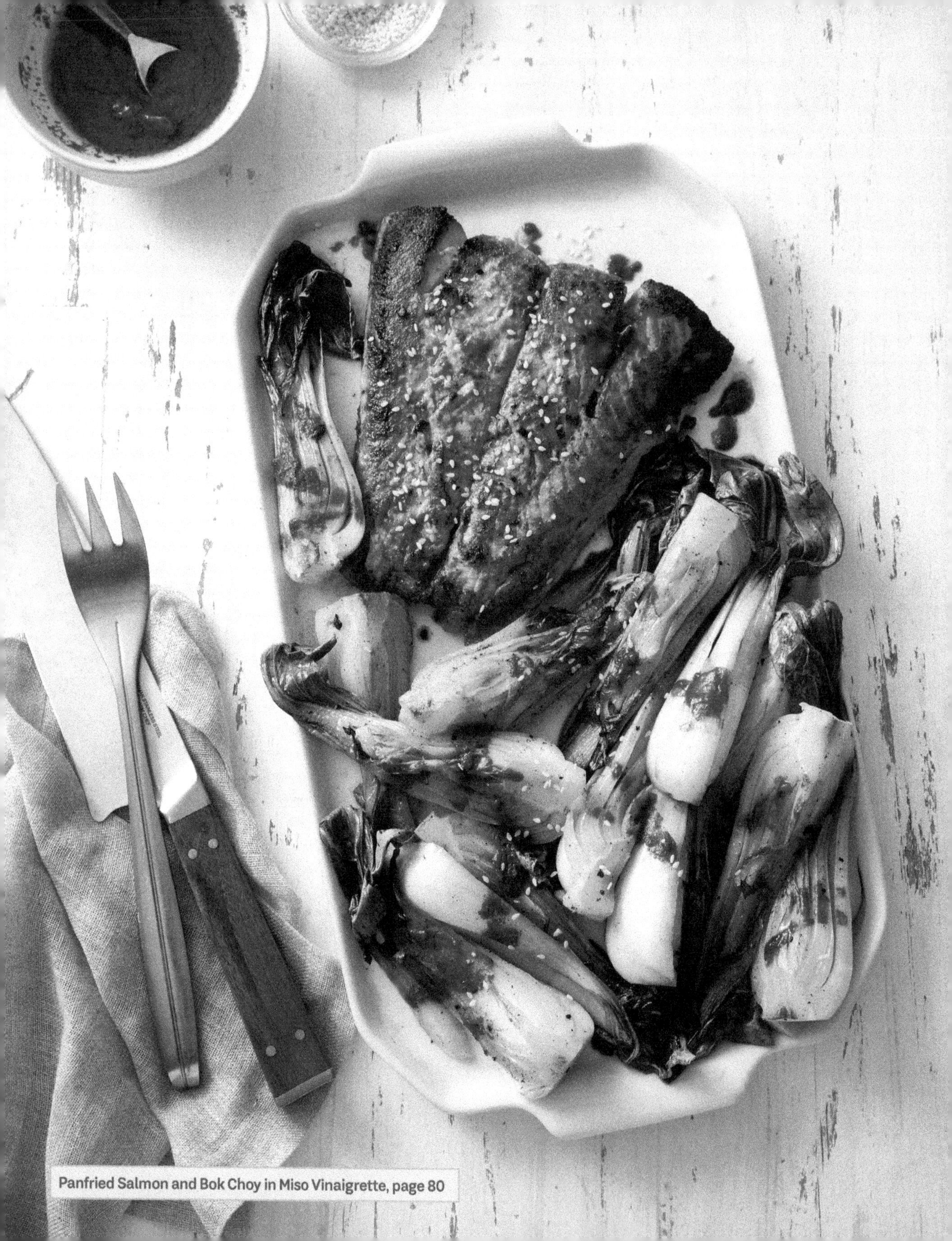

Panfried Salmon and Bok Choy in Miso Vinaigrette, page 80

CHAPTER SIX

Fish and Seafood

PANFRIED SALMON AND BOK CHOY IN MISO VINAIGRETTE

Serves 4 | Prep Time: 10 minutes, plus 30 minutes to marinate | Cook Time: 25 minutes | Dairy-Free, Egg-Free, Gluten-Free, Nut-Free

Bok choy is a wonderful Asian cruciferous vegetable full of antioxidant and anti-inflammatory properties. I love its delicate flavor and unique texture. It can be found in the produce section of most grocery stores, but you can substitute chopped cabbage, halved Brussels sprouts, or broccoli florets, if you desire.

¼ cup miso paste
2 tablespoons rice wine vinegar or dry white wine
6 tablespoons toasted sesame oil, divided
2 teaspoons ground ginger
1 teaspoon red pepper flakes
2 garlic cloves, minced
1 pound wild-caught salmon fillet, skin removed
½ cup avocado or extra-virgin olive oil, divided
8 heads baby bok choy, quartered
2 tablespoons tamari or water
2 tablespoons sesame seeds

1. In a small bowl, combine the miso, vinegar, 2 tablespoons of sesame oil, ginger, red pepper flakes, and garlic and whisk until smooth.

2. In a glass baking dish or resealable storage bag, place the salmon and pour the marinade over it. Refrigerate for at least 30 minutes or up to overnight.

3. To cook the fish, in a large skillet heat 4 tablespoons of avocado oil over medium-high heat. Remove the salmon from the marinade, reserving the liquid, and fry for 3 to 5 minutes per side, until the fish is crispy and golden brown. The time depends on your desired doneness and the thickness of the fish.

4. Transfer the fish to a large platter and keep warm.

5. In the same skillet, add the remaining 4 tablespoons of avocado oil over medium-high heat. Add the bok choy and fry for about 7 minutes, until it is crispy and just tender. Transfer it to the platter with the salmon.

6. Reduce the heat to low. Add the reserved miso marinade and tamari to the oil in the skillet and whisk to combine well. Simmer, uncovered, for 4 to 5 minutes, until slightly thickened. Whisk in the remaining 4 tablespoons of sesame oil until smooth.

7. Serve the salmon and bok choy drizzled with the warm miso vinaigrette and sprinkled with the sesame seeds.

INGREDIENT TIP: Removing skin from raw salmon can be a laborious task, but you can ask your fishmonger to do it for you to save significant time. If you enjoy the flavor of crispy salmon skin, as do I, feel free to leave it on.

Per Serving: Calories: 631; Total Fat: 56g; Total Carbs: 8g; Net Carbs: 5g; Fiber: 3g; Protein: 27g; Sodium: 1334mg; **Macros:** Fat: 80%, Carbs: 3%, Protein: 17%

SEARED COD WITH COCONUT-MUSHROOM SAUCE

Serves 4 | Prep Time: 10 minutes | Cook Time: 20 minutes | Dairy-Free, Egg-Free, Gluten-Free

The rich and creamy mushroom sauce in this dish really dresses up a simple weeknight fish meal. Tamari is a gluten-free version of soy sauce, but you can use miso paste combined with water for a similar flavor, if you don't have tamari on hand.

1 pound cod fillet
½ teaspoon salt
¼ teaspoon freshly ground black pepper
½ cup coconut oil, divided
Grated zest and juice of 1 lime, divided
4 ounces shiitake mushrooms, thinly sliced
2 garlic cloves, minced
1 (13.5-ounce) can full-fat coconut milk
1 teaspoon ground ginger
1 teaspoon red pepper flakes
2 tablespoons tamari (or 1 tablespoon miso paste and 1 tablespoon water)
2 tablespoons toasted sesame oil

1. Cut the cod into four equal pieces and season with salt and pepper.

2. In a large skillet, heat 4 tablespoons of coconut oil over high heat until just before smoking.

3. Add the cod, skin-side up, cover to prevent splattering and sear for 4 to 5 minutes, until it's golden brown. Remove the fish from the skillet, drizzle with the juice of ½ lime, and let rest.

4. In the same skillet, add the remaining 4 tablespoons of coconut oil and heat over medium. Add the mushrooms and sauté for 5 to 6 minutes, until they are just tender. Add the garlic and sauté for 1 minute, until fragrant.

5. Whisk in the coconut milk, ginger, red pepper flakes, tamari, and remaining lime zest and juice and reduce the heat to low. Return the cod to the skillet, skin-side down, cover and simmer for 3 to 4 minutes, until the fish is cooked through.

6. To serve, place the cod on rimmed plates or in shallow bowls and spoon the sauce over the fish. Drizzle with the sesame oil.

Per Serving: Calories: 572; Total Fat: 51g; Total Carbs: 9g; Net Carbs: 7g; Fiber: 2g; Protein: 23g; Sodium: 913mg;
Macros: Fat: 80%, Carbs: 4%, Protein: 16%

THAI-INSPIRED SEAFOOD CHOWDER

Serves 4 | Prep Time: 10 minutes | Cook Time: 15 minutes | Dairy-Free, Egg-Free, Gluten-Free

This easy chowder has a complex flavor but comes together in under 30 minutes for an easy weeknight dinner. You can find Thai green curry paste in the international aisle of most grocery stores.

- 2 tablespoons coconut oil
- 1 red bell pepper, coarsely chopped
- 1 (2-inch) piece fresh ginger, peeled and minced
- 6 garlic cloves, thinly sliced
- 1 jalapeño, finely chopped (seeded for less heat, if preferred)
- 2 teaspoons Thai green curry paste
- 2 (13.5-ounce) cans full-fat coconut milk
- ¼ cup tamari (or 2 tablespoons miso paste and 2 tablespoons water)
- 1 to 2 teaspoons monk fruit extract (optional)
- 8 ounces wild-caught shrimp, peeled and deveined
- 8 ounces cod fillet, skinned and cut into bite-size chunks
- Grated zest and juice of 1 lime
- ½ to 1 cup thinly sliced fresh basil
- Sliced jalapeño, for garnish (optional)

1. In a large stockpot, heat the coconut oil over medium heat. Add the bell pepper, ginger, garlic, and jalapeño and sauté for 4 to 5 minutes, until the vegetables are tender.

2. Add the curry paste and sauté for 1 minute, then add the coconut milk and tamari and whisk to combine well. Stir in the monk fruit extract (if using).

3. Bring the mixture to a boil, reduce the heat to low, add the shrimp and cod, cover and simmer for 3 to 4 minutes, until the seafood is cooked through but not overly done.

4. Remove from the heat and stir in the lime zest and juice and basil. Serve warm, garnished with the jalapeño (if using).

VARIATION TIP: You can substitute chunks of a white flakey fish, such as cod or halibut, for the shrimp if desired. You can use red curry paste or a curry powder blend if that's what you have on hand. Just double the amount of lime zest and juice to produce a similar flavor.

Per Serving: Calories: 512; Total Fat: 41g; Total Carbs: 15g; Net Carbs: 12g; Fiber: 3g; Protein: 27g; Sodium: 1217mg; **Macros:** Fat: 72%, Carbs: 7%, Protein: 21%

SAUTÉED SHRIMP WITH ARUGULA PESTO

Serves 4 | Prep Time: 10 minutes | Cook Time: 5 minutes | Dairy-Free, Egg-Free, Gluten-Free

Traditional pesto is made with basil and pine nuts, which impart a very distinct flavor, but I love using micronutrient-dense arugula and walnuts for a tasty, anti-inflammatory spin on an old favorite. Serve this dish on its own as an appetizer or over spiralized zucchini or Perfect Riced Cauliflower (page 156) for a complete meal.

2 cups packed arugula
1 cup packed whole fresh basil leaves
½ cup chopped walnuts
½ cup freshly shredded Parmesan cheese
2 garlic cloves, peeled
1 teaspoon salt, divided
½ teaspoon freshly ground black pepper
¾ cup extra-virgin olive oil, divided
1 pound wild-caught shrimp, peeled and deveined

1. In a food processor, combine the arugula, basil, walnuts, Parmesan, and garlic and blend until very finely chopped. Add ½ teaspoon of salt and the pepper.

2. With the processor running, stream in ½ cup of olive oil until well blended. If the mixture seems too thick, add warm water, 1 tablespoon at a time, until the texture is smooth and creamy. Set aside.

3. In a large skillet, heat the remaining ¼ cup of olive oil over medium-high heat. Add the shrimp, sprinkle with the remaining ½ teaspoon of salt, and sauté for 3 to 4 minutes, until the shrimp are just pink.

4. Remove from the heat and stir in the pesto to combine well. Serve warm.

MAKE AHEAD: Store the pesto, covered, in the refrigerator for up to one week. I suggest doubling the amount of pesto and keeping half on hand to flavor scrambled eggs, stir into chicken or egg salads, or use as a dip for raw veggies.

Per Serving: Calories: 603; Total Fat: 53g; Total Carbs: 4g; Net Carbs: 3g; Fiber: 1g; Protein: 30g; Sodium: 899mg;
Macros: Fat: 79%, Carbs: 1%, Protein: 20%

SWORDFISH KEBABS WITH MINT CREAM

Serves 4 | Prep Time: 10 minutes | Cook Time: 10 minutes | Dairy-Free, Egg-Free, Gluten-Free

With its fresh and light flavors, this is a wonderful summer evening meal best eaten outside, enjoying the fresh air. The steak-like texture of swordfish holds up well to the grill, but if you are baking these in the oven, a lighter fish such as halibut or cod would work nicely as well. If you are using wooden skewers, be sure to soak them for at least 10 minutes before threading to prevent scorching.

1 (13.5-ounce) can full-fat coconut milk
1 cup packed whole fresh mint leaves
Grated zest and juice of 1 orange
1 teaspoon red pepper flakes
¼ cup extra-virgin olive oil or avocado oil
1 pound swordfish steaks, cut into 2-inch cubes
1 teaspoon salt
½ teaspoon freshly ground black pepper
8 cups mixed greens

1. In a blender or food processor, combine the coconut milk, mint, orange zest and juice, and red pepper flakes and blend well. Stream in the oil and blend until smooth. Place the mixture in the refrigerator until ready to serve.

2. Thread the swordfish cubes onto skewers. Sprinkle with salt and pepper.

3. Heat the grill to medium-high heat. When the grill is very hot, add the skewers and grill for 3 to 4 minutes per side, flipping once, until cooked through.

4. To serve, top 2 cups of salad with 1 kebab and drizzle with the mint cream.

COOKING TIP: To prepare these in the oven, place the kebabs on a slotted broiler pan (to ensure even cooking on all sides and prevent soggy bottoms) and roast in the oven at 450°F for 8 to 10 minutes, turning halfway through the cooking time, until browned and cooked through.

Per Serving: Calories: 491; Total Fat: 38g; Total Carbs: 13g; Net Carbs: 9g; Fiber: 4g; Protein: 26g; Sodium: 764mg; **Macros:** Fat: 70%, Carbs: 9%, Protein: 21%

MEDITERRANEAN POACHED COD

Serves 4 | Prep Time: 5 minutes | Cook Time: 25 minutes | Dairy-Free, Egg-Free, Gluten-Free, Nut-Free

Poaching seafood in a bath of warm olive oil is a cooking style common in many Mediterranean countries. I love the tender and flavorful result, and if you haven't tried it, this is a must! You can use marinated artichokes for even more flavor. I love the buttery flavor of Spanish Manzanilla olives in this dish, but feel free to use any you may have on hand.

- 1 pound cod fillet, cut into 4 equal pieces
- 1 teaspoon salt
- ½ teaspoon freshly ground black pepper
- ½ cup extra-virgin olive oil, divided
- 1 red bell pepper, thinly sliced
- 1 (14-ounce) can artichoke hearts, drained and quartered
- 1 (6-ounce) can large pitted green or black olives, drained and halved
- 4 large garlic cloves, peeled and crushed
- 2 tablespoons chopped fresh rosemary, or 2 teaspoons dried
- ¼ cup white wine vinegar or rice vinegar

1. Sprinkle the cod with salt and pepper.
2. In a large skillet, heat 2 tablespoons of olive oil over medium-high heat. Sear the cod for 1 to 2 minutes per side. Transfer the fish to a serving dish and keep warm.
3. In the same skillet, add the remaining 6 tablespoons of olive oil over medium heat. Add the bell pepper, artichokes, olives, garlic, and rosemary and sauté for 2 to 3 minutes, or until very fragrant.
4. Reduce the heat to low, stir in the vinegar, return the cod to the skillet, cover and poach for 10 to 12 minutes, until the fish is cooked through and the vegetables are tender.
5. Serve the cod and vegetables warm, drizzled with the cooking oil.

Per Serving: Calories: 457; Total Fat: 34g; Total Carbs: 13g; Net Carbs: 9g; Fiber: 4g; Protein: 24g; Sodium: 1690mg; **Macros:** Fat: 67%, Carbs: 12%, Protein: 21%

SNAPPER PICCATA

Serves 4 | Prep Time: 10 minutes | Cook Time: 20 minutes | Egg-Free, Gluten-Free

I love the delicate and slightly sweet taste of red snapper, which pairs nicely with the lemon-butter flavor in this dish. You can also substitute cod or another thin fillet of fish if you can't find snapper. Always aim for grass-fed dairy to ensure the highest quality and anti-inflammatory fats.

¼ cup almond flour
1 teaspoon salt
½ teaspoon freshly ground black pepper
1 pound red snapper fillet, skinned and cut into 4 equal pieces
2 tablespoons extra-virgin olive oil
½ cup (1 stick) unsalted butter, divided
2 tablespoons minced shallot or red onion
2 tablespoons dry white wine
3 tablespoons coarsely chopped capers
Juice of 1 lemon (about 2 tablespoons)
¼ cup chopped parsley

1. In a shallow dish, combine the almond flour, salt, and pepper. Dredge the fish in the flour, shaking off any excess.

2. In a large skillet, heat the olive oil and 2 tablespoons of butter over medium-high heat. Sear the fish for 2 to 3 minutes on each side, until browned and cooked through. Transfer to a serving dish and keep warm.

3. In the same skillet, melt 2 tablespoons of butter. Add the shallot and sauté for 1 to 2 minutes, until just tender. Whisk in the wine, bring to a simmer, then reduce the heat to low. Add the capers and lemon juice and simmer for 1 to 2 minutes.

4. Remove the skillet from the heat and whisk in the remaining 4 tablespoons of butter until melted. Stir in the parsley.

5. To serve, spoon the sauce over each piece of fish.

INGREDIENT TIP: Capers are in the same family as olives and have a wonderfully briny taste. They are often present in tartar sauce and other seafood sauces. Feel free to substitute chopped green olives if you can't find them.

Per Serving: Calories: 281; Total Fat: 23g; Total Carbs: 3g; Net Carbs: 2g; Fiber: 1g; Protein: 16g; Sodium: 677mg; **Macros:** Fat: 74%, Carbs: 3%, Protein: 23%

COCONUT-CRUSTED COD WITH HERB-TARTAR SAUCE

Serves 4 | Prep Time: 15 minutes | Cook Time: 20 minutes | Dairy-Free, Gluten-Free

Loaded with anti-inflammatory omega-3 fatty acids from ground flaxseed, this healthy version of a restaurant favorite is a great addition to any ketogenic diet. You could use another white flakey fish, like flounder or snapper, or even substitute chicken, if preferred.

FOR THE FISH

¼ cup melted coconut oil, divided
¼ cup almond or coconut flour
½ teaspoon salt
¼ teaspoon freshly ground black pepper
½ cup unsweetened coconut flakes
¼ cup ground flaxseed
1 large egg
1 pound cod fillet, skinned and cut into 4 equal pieces

FOR THE SAUCE

½ cup Anti-Inflammatory Mayo (page 148)
2 tablespoons freshly squeezed lemon juice
2 tablespoons coarsely chopped capers
½ teaspoon red pepper flakes (optional)
½ teaspoon salt
¼ teaspoon freshly ground black pepper

TO MAKE THE FISH

1. Preheat the oven to 375°F. Line a baking sheet with aluminum foil and coat with 2 tablespoons of coconut oil.
2. In a shallow bowl, combine the almond flour, salt, and pepper. In a second shallow bowl, combine the coconut flakes and flaxseed. In a third shallow bowl, beat the egg.
3. Dredge each cod piece, one at a time, first in the almond flour, then the egg, and then the coconut-flaxseed mixture, to coat thoroughly. Place the fish on the prepared baking sheet.
4. Drizzle with the remaining 2 tablespoons of coconut oil and bake for 15 to 18 minutes, or until the fish is golden and crispy.

TO MAKE THE SAUCE

5. While the fish cooks, in a small bowl, combine the mayo, lemon juice, capers, red pepper flakes (if using), salt, and pepper and whisk well with a fork. Serve each piece of fish with the sauce.

Per Serving: Calories: 624; Total Fat: 57g; Total Carbs: 7g; Net Carbs: 3g; Fiber: 4g; Protein: 26g; Sodium: 970mg; **Macros:** Fat: 82%, Carbs: 1%, Protein: 17%

SEARED CITRUS SCALLOPS WITH MINT AND BASIL

Serves 4 | Prep Time: 5 minute | Cook Time: 10 minutes | Egg-Free, Gluten-Free, Nut-Free

While they are a bit pricier, larger sea scallops are my preference for this dish over smaller bay scallops. The fresh herbs add not only wonderful flavor but inflammation-reducing properties, so be sure not to leave them out. You can also substitute shrimp or cleaned and sliced squid in this dish. Serve the scallops over Perfect Riced Cauliflower (page 156) or spiralized zucchini.

- 1 pound sea scallops, patted dry
- 1 teaspoon salt, divided
- ½ teaspoon freshly ground black pepper
- ¼ cup extra-virgin olive oil
- 4 tablespoons unsalted butter
- Grated zest and juice of 1 orange
- Grated zest and juice of 1 lemon
- 2 tablespoons chopped fresh mint
- 2 tablespoons chopped fresh basil

1. Sprinkle the scallops with ½ teaspoon of salt and the pepper.

2. In a large skillet, heat the olive oil over medium-high heat. Place the scallops, one by one, into the hot oil and sear for 2 to 3 minutes on each side, or until the scallops are lightly golden. Using a slotted spoon, remove from the skillet and keep warm.

3. Add the butter to the skillet and reduce the heat to medium low. Once the butter has melted, whisk in the citrus zests and juices, mint, basil, and the remaining ½ teaspoon of salt. Cook for 1 minute.

4. Remove from the heat and return the seared scallops to the skillet, tossing to coat them in the butter sauce.

5. Serve the scallops warm, drizzled with sauce.

COOKING TIP: You don't want to overcook the scallops, or they will lose their buttery texture and become chewy. They will continue to cook once removed from the skillet, so be sure to only sear them for the time suggested on each side.

Per Serving: Calories: 338; Total Fat: 26g; Total Carbs: 7g; Net Carbs: 7g; Fiber: <1g; Protein: 20g; Sodium: 844mg; **Macros:** Fat: 69%, Carbs: 7%, Protein: 24%

PANFRIED SHRIMP BALLS OVER GARLICKY GREENS

Serves 4 | Prep Time: 10 minutes, plus 10 minutes to rest | Cook Time: 25 minutes | Dairy-Free

This restaurant-worthy dish takes a little more time to prepare, but it is well worth the effort. Be sure to seek out wild-caught shrimp, as farm-raised seafood is fed a corn-based diet and results in a higher omega-6, pro-inflammatory nutrition profile. Wild-caught seafood contains higher levels of anti-inflammatory omega-3s.

- 1 pound wild-caught shrimp, peeled, deveined, and finely chopped
- ¼ cup coconut or almond flour
- 1 large egg, lightly beaten
- 1 (2-inch) piece fresh ginger, peeled and minced
- ¼ cup minced scallion, green part only, divided
- 1 teaspoon garlic powder
- Grated zest of 1 lime
- ½ teaspoon salt
- ¼ to ½ teaspoon red pepper flakes
- 10 tablespoons extra-virgin olive oil, divided, plus more for frying as needed
- 8 cups kale or spinach, torn into bite-size pieces
- 6 garlic cloves, minced
- ¼ cup soy sauce
- 2 tablespoons rice vinegar
- 2 tablespoons sesame oil

1. In a large bowl, combine the shrimp, coconut flour, egg, ginger, 2 tablespoons of scallion, garlic powder, lime zest, salt, and red pepper flakes, mixing well with a fork. Using your hands, form the shrimp mixture into about a dozen (1-inch) balls and place them on a cutting board or baking sheet lined with parchment paper. Allow to rest for 10 minutes.

2. In a small skillet or saucepan, heat 4 tablespoons of olive oil over medium-high heat. Working in batches of three to four balls, panfry them for 5 to 7 minutes total, carefully turning to brown all sides. Repeat until all the shrimp balls have been fried, adding additional oil with each batch as needed. Keep the shrimp balls warm.

3. In a large skillet, heat 2 tablespoons of olive oil over medium-high heat. Add the greens and sauté for 5 minutes. Add the garlic and sauté for 2 to 4 minutes, or until the greens are wilted.

4. In a small bowl, whisk together the soy sauce, vinegar, and sesame oil.

5. To serve, divide the sautéed greens between plates and top with three shrimp balls drizzled with the sauce.

COOKING TIP: These can be baked in the oven to save cooking time. Coat a baking sheet with ¼ cup of olive oil and space the shrimp balls 1 inch apart in a single layer. Bake at 400°F for 8 to 10 minutes, until lightly browned and set.

Per Serving: Calories: 544; Total Fat: 44g; Total Carbs: 9g; Net Carbs: 4g; Fiber: 5g; Protein: 29g; Sodium: 1361mg; **Macros:** Fat: 73%, Carbs: 6%, Protein: 21%

GREEN TEA POACHED SALMON

Serves 4 | Prep Time: 5 minutes | Cook Time: 40 minutes | Dairy-Free, Egg-Free, Gluten-Free

This dish is a true nutrition powerhouse. The green tea imparts a unique flavor to this slow-cooked, omega-3-rich salmon, and it is full of powerful antioxidants to help reduce inflammation. Most of the cooking time here is hands-off, so this easy dish can come together quickly on a busy weeknight.

- 2 cups water
- 2 tablespoons coconut oil
- 1 (2-inch) piece fresh ginger, peeled and minced, or 2 teaspoons ground ginger
- 4 garlic cloves, very thinly sliced
- 1 teaspoon salt
- 4 green tea bags
- 1 pound wild-caught salmon fillet, skinned and cut into 4 equal pieces
- ¼ cup avocado or extra-virgin olive oil

1. In a medium skillet over medium-high, combine the water, coconut oil, ginger, garlic, and salt. Bring to a boil, cover, reduce the heat to low, and simmer for 10 minutes.
2. Remove from the heat, add the tea bags, cover and steep for 10 minutes.
3. Remove the tea bags from the liquid and discard. Cover and bring to a simmer over medium-low heat. Carefully place the salmon pieces into the simmering liquid, cover and cook for 15 to 18 minutes, until poached through.
4. Using a slotted spoon, remove the salmon pieces from the liquid and serve warm, drizzled with the avocado oil.

Per Serving: Calories: 317; Total Fat: 25g; Total Carbs: 1g; Net Carbs: 1g; Fiber: <1g; Protein: 22g; Sodium: 760mg; **Macros:** Fat: 71%, Carbs: 1%, Protein: 28%

POWER POKE BOWL

Serves 2 | Prep Time: 20 minutes, plus 30 minutes to chill | Dairy-Free, Gluten-Free, Nut-Free

Poke bowls originated in Hawaii and have become very popular across the country, with their blend of flavors and textures and infinite combination possibilities. Many restaurant versions contain higher carbs from rice and sugar-sweetened sauces. Making your own at home takes a bit of prep time but is well worth the effort.

¼ cup tamari
¼ cup sesame oil
1 tablespoon minced fresh ginger, or ½ teaspoon ground ginger
1 to 2 teaspoons red pepper flakes
8 ounces sashimi-grade tuna or smoked salmon, cut into bite-size cubes
¼ cup Anti-Inflammatory Mayo (page 148)
2 tablespoons rice vinegar or freshly squeezed lime juice
1 to 2 teaspoons sriracha or other hot sauce
4 cups mixed greens
¼ cup chopped fresh cilantro or basil
1 avocado, thinly sliced
8 thin slices cucumber
¼ cup thinly sliced scallions, white and green parts
2 teaspoons sesame seeds

1. In a small bowl, whisk together the tamari, sesame oil, ginger, and red pepper flakes. Add the tuna, toss to coat, cover and refrigerate for at least 30 minutes or up to overnight.

2. While the tuna marinates, in a small bowl whisk together the mayo, vinegar, and sriracha. Set aside.

3. To prepare the bowls, divide the salad greens and cilantro between bowls. Top with the avocado, cucumber, and scallions. Add half of the marinated tuna mixture and the liquid to each bowl. Drizzle with the spicy mayonnaise mixture and sesame seeds. Serve immediately.

Per Serving: Calories: 806; Total Fat: 68g; Total Carbs: 16g; Net Carbs: 7g; Fiber: 9g; Protein: 36g; Sodium: 2251mg; **Macros:** Fat: 76%, Carbs: 6%, Protein: 18%

Green Curry with Chicken and Eggplant, page 112

CHAPTER SEVEN

Poultry and Meat

MOROCCAN-INSPIRED GRILLED CHICKEN KEBABS WITH LEMON-TAHINI SAUCE

Serves 4 | Prep Time: 15 minutes, plus 4 hours to marinate and 30 minutes to rest | Cook Time: 15 minutes | Dairy-Free, Egg-Free, Gluten-Free, Nut-Free

The intense flavor in these kebabs is out of this world and full of powerful anti-inflammatory compounds from turmeric, garlic, and red pepper flakes. The creamy dairy-free dipping sauce is a wonderful complement for both flavor and texture. If you don't have tahini on hand, you can substitute almond or cashew butter for similar results. Serve alongside a large tossed salad or roasted veggies with olive oil for a complete meal.

FOR THE SAUCE

¼ cup extra-virgin olive oil
2 tablespoons tahini
1 tablespoon freshly squeezed lemon juice
1 tablespoon tamari
1 garlic clove, pressed or minced

FOR THE CHICKEN KEBABS

¼ cup extra-virgin olive oil
Grated zest and juice of 1 lemon
2 garlic cloves, minced
1 teaspoon ground turmeric
1 teaspoon ground cumin
1 teaspoon paprika
1 teaspoon salt
½ to 1 teaspoon red pepper flakes

TO MAKE THE SAUCE

1. In a small bowl, whisk together the olive oil, tahini, lemon juice, tamari, and garlic until very smooth. (You can also place all ingredients in a glass mason jar, seal it, and shake vigorously to blend.) Refrigerate until ready to use.

TO MAKE THE CHICKEN KEBABS

2. In a small bowl, combine the olive oil, lemon zest and juice, garlic, turmeric, cumin, paprika, salt, red pepper flakes, coriander, and cardamom and mix well.

3. Place the chicken in a resealable plastic bag or glass container with a lid. Add the spice-oil mixture, seal, and toss to coat. Marinate in the refrigerator for 4 hours or up to overnight.

4. To cook, remove the chicken from the refrigerator and let rest at room temperature for at least 30 minutes before grilling. Heat the grill to medium-high heat. If using wooden skewers, fully submerge the skewers in the water for at least 10 minutes before threading to prevent burning.

- ½ teaspoon ground coriander
- ½ teaspoon ground cardamom
- 1 pound boneless, skinless chicken thighs, cut into 2-inch cubes

5. Thread the cubed chicken onto the skewers, dividing evenly. Reserve any leftover marinade for basting while grilling.

6. Grill for 10 to 15 minutes, flipping once, until the chicken is cooked through. Baste the chicken with the reserved marinade as you grill.

7. Remove the skewers from the grill and allow to sit at room temperature for 5 minutes before serving.

8. Serve the chicken with the lemon-tahini sauce.

MAKE AHEAD: The sauce for these makes a great dressing as well. You can double the quantity here and store it in the refrigerator in a sealed container for up to two weeks. If desired, you can thin it out with 1 to 2 tablespoons of olive oil, lemon juice, or water to dress salads.

Per Serving: Calories: 431; Total Fat: 38g; Total Carbs: 5g; Net Carbs: 4g; Fiber: 1g; Protein: 20g; Sodium: 1014mg; **Macros:** Fat: 79%, Carbs: 2%, Protein: 19%

BISON BURGERS IN LETTUCE WRAPS

Serves 4 | Prep Time: 15 minutes | Cook Time: 20 minutes | Egg-Free, Gluten-Free, Nut-Free

With similar flavor to beef, bison tends to be a leaner meat that is almost always free-range and grass-fed. The fats it does have are anti-inflammatory, rather than pro-inflammatory from a corn or grain-based diet. The feta and Middle Eastern spices in these burgers really create a unique and deep flavor—no bun needed!

- 1 pound ground bison
- 4 ounces crumbled sheep's milk feta cheese
- 2 tablespoons extra-virgin olive oil
- 2 teaspoons ground cumin
- 1 teaspoon salt
- 1 teaspoon ground cinnamon
- 1 teaspoon ground ginger
- ½ to 1 teaspoon red pepper flakes
- 4 large Bibb or romaine lettuce leaves, for serving
- 1 cup Spiced Guacamole (page 152), for serving

1. Heat the grill to medium-high heat.
2. In a large bowl, combine the bison, feta, olive oil, cumin, salt, cinnamon, ginger, and red pepper flakes. Using your hands, mix well.
3. Form the mixture into four patties and cook for 5 to 8 minutes on each side, until browned and cooked through to desired doneness.
4. Serve the burgers wrapped in the lettuce leaves and topped with ¼ cup of guacamole per burger.

COOKING TIP: These burgers can also be made in a cast-iron skillet and will be juicy and wonderful. Preheat the oven to 425°F and heat the skillet on the stovetop over high heat. Sear the burgers for 2 to 3 minutes on each side, or until browned. Transfer the skillet to the hot oven to cook the burgers another 5 to 8 minutes, to desired doneness.

Per Serving: Calories: 468; Total Fat: 35g; Total Carbs: 8g; Net Carbs: 3g; Fiber: 5g; Protein: 35g; Sodium: 1400mg; **Macros:** Fat: 67%, Carbs: 3%, Protein: 30%

TURKEY MEATLOAF MUFFINS WITH AVOCADO AIOLI

Makes 12 muffins | Prep Time: 20 minutes | Cook Time: 20 minutes | Dairy-Free, Gluten-Free

On a high-fat ketogenic diet, it is important to focus on heart-healthy unsaturated fats over saturated fats from animal sources for optimal health and sustainability. Here, I use a leaner turkey rather than traditional ground beef and add anti-inflammatory omega-3 fatty acids from olive oil and avocado to keep the macronutrient ratios in check.

½ cup extra-virgin olive oil, divided
1 pound ground turkey
¼ cup almond flour
1 large egg, beaten
1 teaspoon dried oregano
1 teaspoon garlic powder
2 teaspoons salt, divided
1 teaspoon freshly ground black pepper, divided
2 tablespoons no-sugar-added tomato paste
2 very ripe avocados, pitted and peeled
1 tablespoon freshly squeezed lemon juice
2 garlic cloves, minced

1. Preheat the oven to 350°F and coat a 12-cup muffin tin with 2 tablespoons of olive oil.

2. In a large bowl, combine the turkey, almond flour, egg, oregano, garlic powder, 1 teaspoon of salt, 2 tablespoons of olive oil, and ½ teaspoon of pepper, combining well with a fork.

3. In a small bowl, combine the tomato paste and 2 tablespoons of olive oil and whisk until well combined.

4. Place about ¼ cup of the meatloaf mixture into each muffin cup. Brush the top of each meatloaf with the tomato mixture and bake for 18 to 20 minutes, until cooked through.

5. While the muffins cook, place the avocado in a medium bowl and mash well with a fork. Add the lemon juice, garlic, the remaining 1 teaspoon of salt, the remaining ½ teaspoon of pepper, and the remaining 4 tablespoons of olive oil and whisk until well combined.

6. Serve the muffins warm topped with the avocado aioli.

VARIATION TIP: The avocado aioli can be thinned out with additional lemon juice or vinegar for a delicious salad dressing. I suggest making extra and storing in the refrigerator for a quick weekday lunch of a simple salad topped with protein.

Per Serving (2 muffins): Calories: 421; Total Fat: 38g; Total Carbs: 7g; Net Carbs: 3g; Fiber: 4g; Protein: 16g; Sodium: 846mg;
Macros: Fat: 81%, Carbs: 4%, Protein: 15%

SLOW-COOKER PUMPKIN CHICKEN

Serves 4 | Prep Time: 5 minutes | Cook Time: 6 hours | Dairy-Free, Egg-Free, Gluten-Free

Pumpkin is a wonderful, nutrient-dense starchy vegetable full of antioxidants, vitamin A, and fiber. Since it is higher in carbohydrates, it is often excluded on a ketogenic diet. In this dish, a little goes a long way, and using the healthy fat–rich seeds from this nutritious vegetable allows for wonderful flavor without compromising keto macro ratios.

- 1 pound boneless, skinless chicken thighs
- ½ cup unsweetened canned pumpkin puree
- ½ cup full-fat canned coconut milk
- ½ cup chicken broth or water
- 2 teaspoons ground cumin
- 1 teaspoon ground cinnamon
- 1 teaspoon ground ginger
- 1 teaspoon salt
- ½ teaspoon ground cloves
- ¼ cup extra-virgin olive oil
- ¼ cup shelled pumpkin seeds

1. Place the chicken in the pot of a slow cooker.
2. In a small bowl, whisk together the pumpkin puree, coconut milk, broth, cumin, cinnamon, ginger, salt, and cloves and pour the mixture over the chicken, stirring to coat.
3. Turn the slow cooker to the low setting and cook for 4 to 6 hours, or until the chicken is very tender.
4. Before serving, in a small skillet heat the olive oil over medium heat. Add the pumpkin seeds and panfry for 3 to 4 minutes, until lightly browned but not burned. Serve the chicken in the pumpkin sauce drizzled with the seeds and oil.

Per Serving: Calories: 363; Total Fat: 30g; Total Carbs: 6g; Net Carbs: 4g; Fiber: 2g; Protein: 22g; Sodium: 875mg; **Macros:** Fat: 74%, Carbs: 2%, Protein: 24%

BEEF STROGANOFF MEATBALLS OVER ZOODLES

Serves 4 | Prep Time: 15 minutes | Cook Time: 30 minutes | Gluten-Free

Here's a keto-friendly spin on a classic comfort dish that the whole family will love. This is a great way to use leftover Cream of Mushroom and Fennel Soup, which keeps well in the freezer to have on hand for other casserole dishes.

- 1 pound grass-fed ground beef or bison
- ¼ cup, plus 2 tablespoons almond flour, divided
- 2 tablespoons minced onion
- 1 teaspoon salt
- 1 teaspoon dried thyme
- ½ teaspoon garlic powder
- ¼ teaspoon freshly ground black pepper
- 1 large egg, beaten
- ¼ cup extra-virgin olive oil
- 2 cups Cream of Mushroom and Fennel Soup (page 54)
- ⅓ cup sour cream
- 4 cups raw spiralized zucchini

1. In a large bowl, combine the ground beef, ¼ cup of almond flour, onion, salt, thyme, garlic powder, and pepper and mix well with a fork. Mix in the egg until well combined. Using your hands, form the mixture into 1-inch round meatballs and set aside.

2. In a shallow dish, place the remaining 2 tablespoons of almond flour and roll the meatballs in the flour.

3. In a large skillet, heat the olive oil over medium-high heat. Add the meatballs and sauté for 6 to 8 minutes, turning to brown on all sides.

4. Add the soup and bring to a boil. Reduce the heat to low, cover and cook for 15 to 20 minutes, until the meatballs are cooked through.

5. Remove from the heat and stir in the sour cream until well blended. To serve, top the raw zucchini noodles with the hot meatballs and sauce and toss to combine.

Per Serving: Calories: 580; Total Fat: 46g; Total Carbs: 13g; Net Carbs: 10g; Fiber: 3g; Protein: 30g; Sodium: 1202mg; **Macros:** Fat: 71%, Carbs: 8%, Protein: 21%

GREEK STUFFED CHICKEN BREASTS

Serves 4 | Prep Time: 20 minutes | Cook Time: 50 minutes, plus 10 minutes to rest | Egg-Free, Gluten-Free, Nut-Free

Lean proteins, such as chicken breast, are usually avoided on ketogenic diets as their high protein-to-fat ratio can push macro breakdowns out of the ideal range. When you pair lean proteins with the delicious anti-inflammatory monounsaturated fats in olives and olive oil, you have a winning combination that not only helps achieve health goals, but is delicious and satiating.

½ cup extra-virgin olive oil, divided
2 boneless, skinless chicken breasts (about 6 ounces each)
4 ounces frozen spinach, thawed and well drained
4 ounces crumbled sheep's milk feta cheese
2 tablespoons chopped pitted Kalamata olives
1 teaspoon salt, divided
1 teaspoon freshly ground black pepper, divided
½ teaspoon garlic powder
½ teaspoon dried oregano
¼ teaspoon red pepper flakes
Grated zest and juice of 1 lemon

1. Preheat the oven to 375°F.

2. In a small deep baking dish, drizzle 1 tablespoon of olive oil and swirl to coat bottom.

3. Make a deep incision about 3 to 4 inches long along the length of each chicken breast, saving 1 inch on each end, to create a pocket. Using your knife or fingers, carefully increase the size of the pocket without cutting through the chicken breast. Each breast will look like a change purse with an opening at the top.

4. In a medium bowl, combine the spinach, feta, olives, 2 tablespoons of olive oil, ½ teaspoon of salt, ½ teaspoon of pepper, garlic powder, oregano, and red pepper flakes and combine well with a fork.

5. Stuff half of the filling into the pocket of each chicken breast, stuffing down to fully fill the pocket. Press the opening together with your fingers. Use a couple of toothpicks to thread it together, if desired.

6. In a medium skillet, heat 2 tablespoons of olive oil over medium-high heat. Add the chicken breasts and sear for 3 to 4 minutes per side, being careful to not let too much filling escape, until browned. Transfer the chicken, incision-side up, to the prepared baking dish. Scrape up any filling that fell out in the skillet and add it to baking dish. Cover with aluminum foil and bake for 30 to 40 minutes, until the chicken is cooked through.

7. Remove from the oven and let rest, covered, for 10 minutes. Meanwhile, whisk together the remaining 3 tablespoons of olive oil, the lemon zest and juice, the remaining ½ teaspoon of salt, and the remaining ½ teaspoon of pepper.

8. To serve, cut each chicken breast in half, width-wise. Serve half a chicken breast drizzled with the lemon oil.

INGREDIENT TIP: You can use store-bought olive tapenade in place of the chopped olives for more intense flavor and convenience. Look for brands that use olive oil rather than canola or soybean oil.

Per Serving: Calories: 431; Total Fat: 36g; Total Carbs: 4g; Net Carbs: 3g; Fiber: 1g; Protein: 24g; Sodium: 1037mg; **Macros:** Fat: 75%, Carbs: 3%, Protein: 22%

CHICKEN MARGHERITA

Serves 4 | Prep Time: 5 minutes | Cook Time: 25 minutes | Gluten-Free, Nut-Free

This has all the classic flavors of my favorite simple and fresh pizza, without all the carbs! For a vegetarian version, substitute portabella mushroom caps or thinly sliced eggplant for the chicken, but don't skimp on the fresh mozzarella and basil, as they really make this simple dish shine.

½ cup extra-virgin olive oil, divided
1 pound chicken breasts, cut into 4 (½-inch-thick) slices
1 teaspoon salt, divided
½ teaspoon freshly ground black pepper, divided
¼ cup Anti-Inflammatory Mayo (page 148)
2 tablespoons no-sugar-added tomato paste
4 ounces fresh mozzarella, cut into 8 (½-inch-thick) slices
8 large whole fresh basil leaves

1. Preheat the oven to 375°F.
2. In a glass baking dish, drizzle 2 tablespoons of olive oil and swirl to coat the bottom.
3. Place the chicken in the baking dish in a single layer and sprinkle with ½ teaspoon of salt and ¼ teaspoon of pepper.
4. In a small bowl, whisk together the mayo, tomato paste, and 2 tablespoons of olive oil. Spread the sauce mixture evenly over each chicken slice and top each piece with two slices of mozzarella.
5. Cover with aluminum foil and bake for 18 to 20 minutes, until the chicken is cooked through. Remove the foil and bake for 5 to 6 minutes, or until the cheese is slightly browned on top.
6. Serve the chicken pieces warm, each topped with two basil leaves and 1 tablespoon of the remaining olive oil. Season with the remaining ½ teaspoon of salt and ¼ teaspoon of pepper.

Per Serving: Calories: 583; Total Fat: 50g; Total Carbs: 2g; Net Carbs: 1g; Fiber: 1g; Protein: 31g; Sodium: 804mg; **Macros:** Fat: 77%, Carbs: 2%, Protein: 21%

ITALIAN WEDDING SOUP WITH KALE

Serves 4 | Prep Time: 15 minutes | Cook Time: 20 minutes | Gluten-Free, Nut-Free

My first time trying Italian wedding soup was when a dear chef friend of mine brought me dinner after having my first child. I was instantly hooked! Many restaurant or store-bought canned versions contain orzo or pearled pasta, and lack all the wonderful flavor of a simple homemade stew. If you are used to bland canned soup, you are in for a treat with this hearty and filling stew.

- 8 ounces grass-fed ground beef
- 8 ounces ground pork
- ¼ cup chopped fresh parsley
- ¼ cup, plus 2 tablespoons freshly grated Parmesan cheese, divided
- 2 tablespoons minced onion
- 2 garlic cloves, minced
- 1 teaspoon salt
- ½ teaspoon freshly ground black pepper
- 8 cups chicken stock
- ½ cup extra-virgin olive oil
- 4 cups torn, stemmed kale
- 2 large eggs

1. In a large bowl, combine the beef, pork, parsley, ¼ cup of Parmesan, onion, garlic, salt, and pepper and combine with a fork. Using your hands, form the mixture into 1-inch meatballs.

2. In a large stock pot over high heat, combine the chicken stock and olive oil and bring to a boil. Add the kale and carefully drop the meatballs into the pot. Reduce the heat to low, cover and simmer for 8 to 10 minutes, until the meatballs are cooked through.

3. In a small bowl, whisk together the eggs and the remaining 2 tablespoons of Parmesan. Using a large spoon, stir the stew in a circular direction and slowly stream in the egg and cheese mixture. Continue to cook, stirring over low heat, for 1 minute, or until the egg is cooked through. Serve warm.

Per Serving: Calories: 597; Total Fat: 49g; Total Carbs: 3g; Net Carbs: 2g; Fiber: 1g; Protein: 37g; Sodium: 1856mg;
Macros: Fat: 74%, Carbs: 1%, Protein: 25%

GROUND BISON CHILES RELLENOS WITH RANCHERO SAUCE

Serves 4 | Prep Time: 30 minutes | Cook Time: 1 hour 35 minutes | Egg-Free, Gluten-Free, Nut-Free

This recipe adds anti-inflammatory monounsaturated fats from olive oil to keep macro ratios ketogenic. The fresh homemade ranchero sauce is full of antioxidant-rich vegetables and flavor. Don't skip the pumpkin seed garnish, as it adds a delicious crunch and plenty of omega-3s.

4 large whole poblano chiles
2 ripe tomatoes, quartered
1 red bell pepper, quartered
1 small jalapeño, stemmed and halved
1 small red onion, quartered
8 garlic cloves, peeled
½ cup extra-virgin olive oil, divided
2 teaspoons salt, divided
8 ounces ground bison
1 teaspoon ground cumin
1 teaspoon ground coriander
1 teaspoon chili powder
1 teaspoon fennel seed
1 teaspoon garlic powder
4 ounces frozen spinach, thawed and well drained
4 ounces goat cheese
1 small bunch fresh cilantro, leaves only
Grated zest and juice of 1 lime

1. Preheat the oven to 425°F.

2. Line a baking sheet with aluminum foil and arrange the chiles in a single layer on it. Roast for 20 to 25 minutes, or until the chiles are just tender and wilted but not blackened. Remove from the oven and allow to cool on the foil, but keep the oven on.

3. Meanwhile, in a large glass baking dish, place the tomatoes, bell pepper, jalapeño, onion, and garlic. Drizzle with 4 tablespoons of olive oil and 1 teaspoon of salt and toss to coat. Roast for 40 to 45 minutes, stirring once halfway through, until the vegetables are soft and lightly browned. Remove from the oven and let cool, but keep the oven on.

4. Meanwhile, in a medium skillet, heat 2 tablespoons of olive oil over medium-high heat. Add the bison and cook, stirring occasionally, for 4 to 5 minutes, until browned. Add the cumin, coriander, chili powder, fennel, garlic powder, and the remaining 1 teaspoon of salt. Mix well and sauté for 1 to 2 minutes. Remove from the heat and stir in the spinach and goat cheese, mixing well.

5. To make the ranchero sauce, transfer the cooled roasted vegetables to a blender or food processor. Add the cilantro and lime zest and juice and blend until smooth. Set aside.

- 1 large avocado, thinly sliced, for serving
- 1 lime, cut into wedges, for serving
- 2 tablespoons roasted pumpkin seeds, for serving

6. To stuff the chiles, carefully cut a slit in each one from the stem to the end and, using your fingers, gently remove the seeds and membrane. Stuff each chile with the bison and spinach mixture.

7. Spread half of the sauce on the bottom of a glass baking dish (you can use the same dish used to roast the vegetables). Place the chiles in a single layer on top, then spread the remaining sauce evenly over the chiles. Drizzle them with the remaining 2 tablespoons of olive oil and cover with foil. Bake for 20 minutes. Remove the foil and bake another 5 minutes, or until bubbly. Serve warm with the avocado, lime wedges, and pumpkin seeds.

VARIATION TIP: You can substitute grass-fed ground beef for the bison in this recipe if desired. However, bison tends to be a bit leaner and lower in saturated fat than beef, while having a very similar flavor.

Per Serving: Calories: 605; Total Fat: 50g; Total Carbs: 22g; Net Carbs: 13g; Fiber: 9g; Protein: 24g; Sodium: 1390mg; **Macros:** Fat: 74%, Carbs: 10%, Protein: 16%

ZOODLES BOLOGNESE

Serves 4 | Prep Time: 5 minutes | Cook Time: 20 minutes | Egg-Free, Gluten-Free, Nut-Free

Spaghetti with meat sauce is a simple comfort meal that makes for an easy weeknight dinner. This variation uses my no-sugar-added marinara sauce and zucchini noodles in place of the pasta for an anti-inflammatory ketogenic meal.

- 2 tablespoons extra-virgin olive oil
- 1 pound grass-fed ground beef or bison
- 1 teaspoon salt
- ½ teaspoon freshly ground black pepper
- 4 cups Easy Marinara Sauce (page 153)
- 4 cups raw spiralized zucchini
- Freshly shredded Parmesan cheese, for serving

1. In a skillet, heat the olive oil over medium heat. Add the beef, salt, and pepper and sauté for 4 to 5 minutes, until the beef is browned. Add the marinara sauce and bring to a simmer. Reduce the heat to low, cover, and cook for 15 minutes.

2. Serve the meat sauce over the zucchini noodles, tossing to coat, and garnish with Parmesan.

COOKING TIP: If you are short on time, you can use a store-bought sauce, but you will need to mix in 2 tablespoons of olive oil per serving (½ cup for 4 servings) to keep the ketogenic ratio.

Per Serving: Calories: 526; Total Fat: 38g; Total Carbs: 22g; Net Carbs: 16g; Fiber: 6g; Protein: 27g; Sodium: 1707mg; **Macros:** Fat: 65%, Carbs: 14%, Protein: 21%

SLOW-COOKER SPICED CHICKEN

Serves 8 | Prep Time: 15 minutes | Cook Time: 5 hours | Egg-Free, Gluten-Free

Intensely rich and flavorful, this is a great simple meal to make for eating leftovers throughout the week. If you are only cooking for one or two, freeze leftover portions in individual containers to have on hand during busy weeks. Serve over Perfect Riced Cauliflower (page 156) or sautéed spinach.

½ cup (1 stick) unsalted butter
½ onion, finely chopped
1 (2-inch) piece fresh ginger, peeled and finely chopped
6 garlic cloves, minced
2 teaspoons salt
1 tablespoon garam masala
1 teaspoon ground turmeric
½ to 1 teaspoon red pepper flakes
1 (13.5-ounce) can full-fat coconut milk
2 tablespoons no-sugar-added tomato paste
2 pounds boneless, skinless chicken breasts, cut into 1-inch pieces
¼ cup chopped fresh cilantro, basil, or mint, for serving

1. In a large skillet or saucepan, melt the butter over medium heat. Add the onion and ginger and sauté for 5 minutes, until the onion is softened. Add the garlic, salt, garam masala, turmeric, and red pepper flakes and sauté for 2 minutes, until fragrant. Add the coconut milk and tomato paste and whisk to combine. Bring the mixture to a simmer, then remove from the heat.

2. Place the chicken pieces in the pot of a slow cooker. Pour the sauce mixture over the chicken, cover, and cook on low for 4 to 5 hours, or until the chicken is very tender.

3. Serve the chicken and sauce mixture garnished with the cilantro.

Per Serving: Calories: 326; Total Fat: 23g; Total Carbs: 5g; Net Carbs: 4g; Fiber: 1g; Protein: 26g; Sodium: 739mg;
Macros: Fat: 63%, Carbs: 5%, Protein: 32%

SLOW-COOKER PULLED PORK

Serves 6 to 8 | Prep Time: 10 minutes | Cook Time: 6 hours | Dairy-Free, Egg-Free, Gluten-Free, Nut-Free

This is an easy alternative to high-sugar versions of barbecued pork. Use leftovers throughout the week atop a lunchtime salad or as a sandwich with a Keto Sandwich Round (page 146). Serve with a side of Classic Coleslaw (page 59) for a complete summertime meal.

½ cup extra-virgin olive oil, divided
2 pounds boneless pork loin, untrimmed and cut into 4 to 6 large chunks
6 garlic cloves, crushed with the back of a knife
2 teaspoons ground cumin
1½ teaspoons salt
1 teaspoon smoked paprika
1 teaspoon red pepper flakes
¼ cup red wine vinegar or apple cider vinegar

1. In the pot of a slow cooker, heat 2 tablespoons of olive oil over high heat.

2. Place the pork pieces in a single layer in the oil. Add the garlic, cumin, salt, paprika, and red pepper flakes and stir to coat the meat. Cook the pork for 1 to 2 minutes on each side, until browned, and reduce the heat to low. Add the vinegar, cover, and cook on low for 6 hours, or until the pork is very tender.

3. Using a slotted spoon, transfer the pork to a large bowl and shred with two forks. Return the pork to the slow cooker, add the remaining 6 tablespoons of olive oil, and toss to combine with the cooking liquid.

Per Serving: Calories: 426; Total Fat: 31g; Total Carbs: 2g; Net Carbs: 2g; Fiber: <1g; Protein: 33g; Sodium: 663mg; **Macros:** Fat: 65%, Carbs: 4%, Protein: 31%

SPICE-RUBBED ROASTED PORK WITH CILANTRO PESTO

Serves 8 | Prep Time: 15 minutes, plus 15 minutes to rest | Cook Time: 1 hour | Dairy-Free, Egg-Free, Gluten-Free, Nut-Free

This recipe packs a ton of flavor and makes enough for leftovers throughout the week. You can easily double the recipe if you're feeding a crowd. Serve any leftover pork atop a bed of mixed greens with the pesto drizzled over the top.

¾ cup extra-virgin olive oil, divided
2 teaspoons ground cumin
1 teaspoon chili powder
1 teaspoon garlic powder
2 teaspoons salt, divided
2 pounds untrimmed pork loin roast
1 cup packed whole fresh cilantro leaves
2 garlic cloves, peeled and smashed
Grated zest and juice of 1 lime

1. Preheat the oven to 375°F.

2. In a small bowl, combine 2 tablespoons of olive oil, cumin, chili powder, garlic powder, and 1 teaspoon of salt to form a paste. Rub the pork with the seasoning and let it sit for 15 minutes.

3. In a large ovenproof skillet or Dutch oven, heat 2 tablespoons of oil over medium-high heat. Add the pork and cook for 3 to 4 minutes per side, until browned.

4. Cover and roast for 40 to 45 minutes, until the internal temperature reaches 150°F. Remove the roast from the oven, and let sit, covered, for 10 minutes to bring the internal temperature to 165°F before slicing.

5. To make the pesto, in the bowl of a food processor or blender, place the cilantro, garlic, and lime zest and juice and blend until well chopped. With the processor running, stream in the remaining 8 tablespoons of olive oil and blend until smooth.

6. Serve the pork drizzled with the cilantro pesto.

MAKE AHEAD: The flavorful cilantro pesto is great mixed in with scrambled eggs or as a sauce on simple grilled fish. I suggest doubling the recipe to have on hand in the refrigerator. Pesto will last in a sealed container for up to two weeks.

Per Serving: Calories: 374; Total Fat: 30g; Total Carbs: 2g; Net Carbs: 2g; Fiber: <1g; Protein: 24g; Sodium: 655mg;
Macros: Fat: 72%, Carbs: 2%, Protein: 26%

GREEN CURRY WITH CHICKEN AND EGGPLANT

Serves 4 | Prep Time: 10 minutes | Cook Time: 25 minutes | Dairy-Free, Egg-Free, Gluten-Free

Curries, which originated in the Indian subcontinent, are a quick and easy way to use extra produce or protein at the end of the week and pack a big flavor punch. Remember that anti-inflammatory turmeric can be bitter to some, so use less if you are not accustomed to its unique flavor. Serve this Thai-inspired curry over Perfect Riced Cauliflower (page 156).

¼ cup coconut oil
1 pound boneless, skinless chicken thighs, cut into 1-inch pieces
½ onion, chopped
2 cups cubed eggplant
4 garlic cloves, minced
2 teaspoons green curry paste
1 teaspoon ground turmeric
1 teaspoon salt
½ to 1 teaspoon red pepper flakes (optional)
2 (13.5-ounce) cans full-fat coconut milk
1 to 2 teaspoons monk fruit extract (optional)
Grated zest of 1 lime (reserve lime for serving)
¼ cup thinly sliced fresh basil, mint, or cilantro

1. In a large stockpot or skillet, heat the coconut oil over medium-high heat. Add the chicken, onion, and eggplant and sauté for 5 to 6 minutes, or until the chicken is browned and the vegetables are just tender.

2. Stir in the garlic, curry paste, turmeric, salt, and red pepper flakes (if using) and sauté for 2 minutes, until very fragrant.

3. Add the coconut milk, monk fruit extract (if using), and lime zest and bring to a boil. Reduce the heat to low, cover, and simmer for 15 to 20 minutes. Serve warm, garnished with lime slices and the basil.

VARIATION TIP: This recipe uses chicken and eggplant, a flavor combination that I love, but feel free to substitute another nonstarchy vegetable you may have on hand, such as cauliflower, broccoli, green beans, or asparagus.

Per Serving: Calories: 603; Total Fat: 54g; Total Carbs: 15g; Net Carbs: 11g; Fiber: 4g; Protein: 22g; Sodium: 898mg;
Macros: Fat: 81%, Carbs: 4%, Protein: 15%

HERBY ROASTED CHICKEN

Serves 4 to 6 | Prep Time: 15 minutes | Cook Time: 1 hour, plus 10 minutes to rest | Dairy-Free, Egg-Free, Gluten-Free, Nut-Free

Roasted chicken is the quintessential homemade meal and so much easier to prepare than most people think! Roast up a chicken or two on Sunday and you'll have enough for a meal as well as lunches throughout the week.

1 (3- to 4-pound) whole chicken
½ cup extra-virgin olive oil, divided
2 teaspoons salt, divided
1 teaspoon freshly ground black pepper, divided
¼ cup chopped fresh rosemary
8 garlic cloves, coarsely chopped
2 tablespoons fresh thyme

1. Preheat the oven to 450°F.

2. Pat the chicken dry with paper towels and rub the outside with 2 tablespoons of olive oil, 1 teaspoon of salt, and ½ teaspoon of pepper.

3. In a small bowl, combine the remaining 6 tablespoons of olive oil, the rosemary, garlic, thyme, the remaining 1 teaspoon of salt, and the remaining ½ teaspoon of pepper.

4. Loosen the skin over the breasts and thighs of the chicken by cutting a small incision in the skin and sticking one or two fingers inside to pull the skin away from the meat without removing it.

5. Stuff a quarter of the oil mixture under the skin of each breast and each thigh and place the chicken, breast-side up, in a roasting pan or large glass baking dish.

6. Roast the chicken for 50 to 60 minutes, or until the internal temperature reaches 165°F and the juices run clear. Remove from the oven and let the chicken rest for 10 minutes before slicing to serve.

VARIATION TIP: Toss leftover shredded chicken with Anti-Inflammatory Mayo (page 148) and chopped celery or capers for an easy chicken salad.

Per Serving: Calories: 611; Total Fat: 48g; Total Carbs: 3g; Net Carbs: 2g; Fiber: 1g; Protein: 42g; Sodium: 1304mg;
Macros: Fat: 71%, Carbs: 2%, Protein: 27%

MOZZARELLA-STUFFED BURGERS

Serves 4 | Prep Time: 5 minutes | Cook Time: 15 minutes | Gluten-Free

You're in for a surprise biting into these burgers. Filled with gooey mozzarella and packed with flavor, they are sure to be a new favorite way to enjoy a classic. The spinach adds a punch of antioxidant micronutrients, but you can omit it and opt for a side salad or sautéed spinach instead.

- 1 pound grass-fed ground beef or bison
- 4 ounces frozen spinach, thawed and well drained
- 2 tablespoons chopped basil
- 1 teaspoon garlic powder
- 1 teaspoon salt
- ½ teaspoon freshly ground black pepper
- 1 (4-ounce) ball fresh mozzarella cheese, quartered
- 4 Keto Sandwich Rounds (page 146)
- ½ cup Lemon-Turmeric Aioli (page 149), for serving

1. Heat the grill to medium-high heat.
2. In a large bowl, combine the beef, spinach, basil, garlic powder, salt, and pepper and, using your hands, mix well.
3. Form into four balls. Sticking your thumb into the center of each ball, create a pocket and stuff one piece of mozzarella into the center, then form into a patty shape.
4. Place the burgers on the grill and cook for 5 to 8 minutes per side, until browned and cooked through to your desired doneness.
5. Serve the burgers on the sandwich rounds, each topped with 2 tablespoons of aioli.

COOKING TIP: To prepare on the stovetop, heat a large cast-iron or other heavy-duty skillet over medium-high heat. Add the burgers, cover, and cook 5 to 6 minutes on each side, or until they are cooked through to the desired doneness.

Per Serving (1 burger, keto round, and 2 tablespoons aioli): Calories: 909; Total Fat: 78g; Total Carbs: 8g; Net Carbs: 5g; Fiber: 3g; Protein: 40g; Sodium: 1431mg;
Macros: Fat: 77%, Carbs: 5%, Protein: 18%

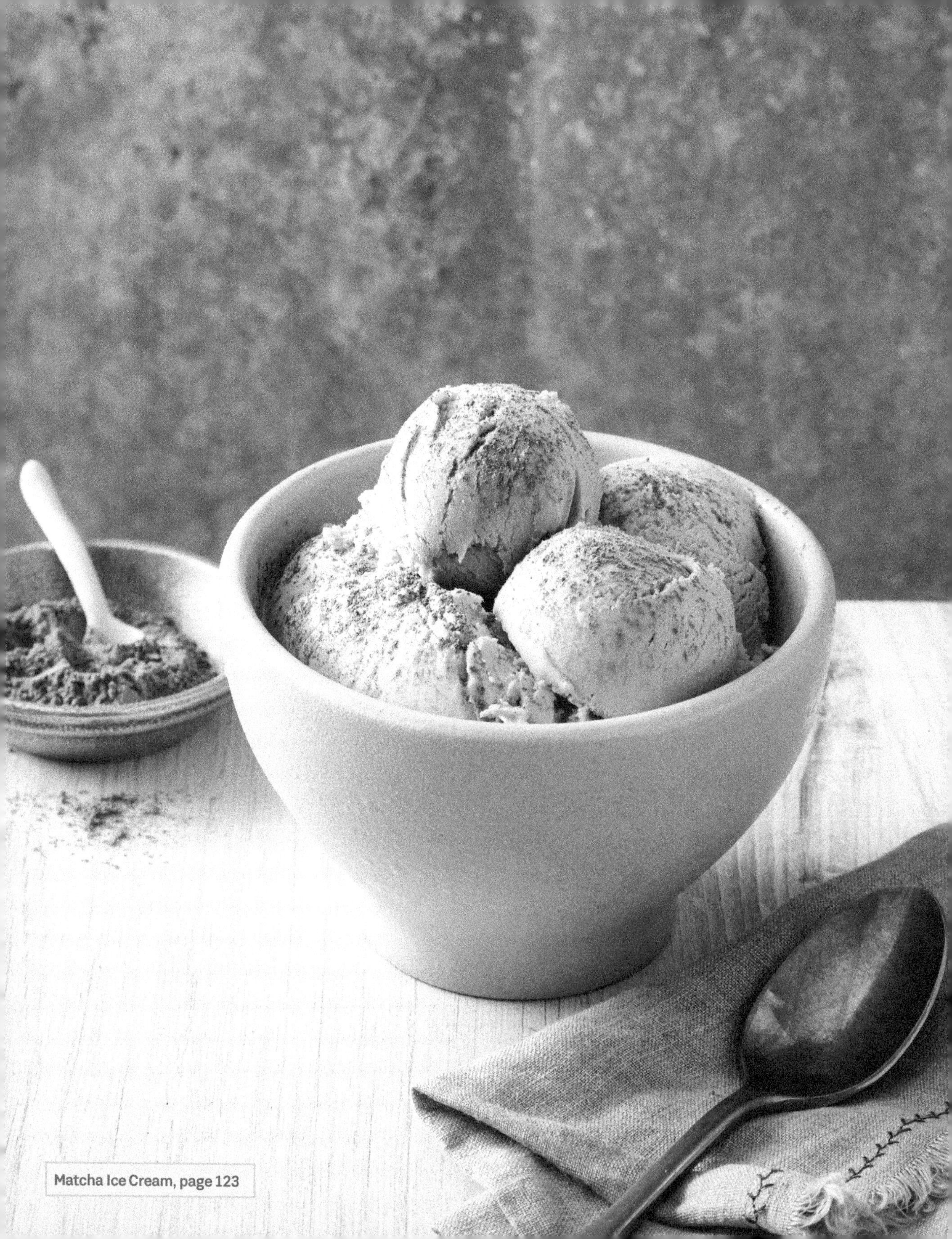

Matcha Ice Cream, page 123

CHAPTER EIGHT

Desserts

MEXICAN CHOCOLATE-INSPIRED PUDDING

Serves 4 | Prep Time: 10 minutes, plus 30 minutes to chill | Dairy-Free, Egg-Free, Gluten-Free, Vegetarian

Just when you thought you couldn't come up with yet another way to enjoy the delicious anti-inflammatory fats in avocados, dessert comes to the rescue. It may sound different, but the creamy avocado creates an out-of-this-world texture and flavor. The addition of cinnamon and cayenne is inspired by Mexican chocolate and adds an anti-inflammatory boost.

2 avocados, halved and pitted
¼ cup unsweetened cocoa powder
¼ cup full-fat canned coconut milk, plus more if needed
2 teaspoons vanilla extract
2 teaspoons monk fruit extract
1 teaspoon ground cinnamon
¼ teaspoon ground cayenne pepper
¼ teaspoon salt

1. Using a spoon, scoop the avocado into a blender or tall narrow container (if using an immersion blender). Add the cocoa, coconut milk, vanilla, monk fruit extract, cinnamon, cayenne, and salt and blend well until smooth and creamy. If the mixture is too thick, add additional coconut milk, 1 tablespoon at a time, until the desired consistency is reached.

2. Cover and refrigerate for at least 30 minutes before serving.

VARIATION TIP: You can use heavy whipping cream or half-and-half in place of coconut milk for a more subtle flavor.

Per Serving: Calories: 159; Total Fat: 14g; Total Carbs: 12g; Net Carbs: 5g; Fiber: 7g; Protein: 3g; Sodium: 156mg; **Macros:** Fat: 79%, Carbs: 13%, Protein: 8%

90-SECOND LAVA CAKE

Serves 1 | Prep Time: 5 minutes | Cook Time: 1 to 2 minutes | Egg-Free, Gluten-Free, Vegetarian

A decadent treat to satisfy any sweet tooth, this microwavable treat for one is there for you when a craving strikes. You can find 100 percent cocoa dark chocolate at most grocery stores, and it has a richer flavor than regular unsweetened baking chocolate. I love the intense chocolate flavor here, but feel free to adjust the sweetener to your taste. This is delicious served warm with whipped cream or a scoop of Matcha Ice Cream (page 123).

- 1 ounce unsweetened dark chocolate (100 percent cocoa), coarsely chopped
- 1 tablespoon unsalted butter
- 1 tablespoon heavy whipping cream
- ¼ teaspoon vanilla extract
- 2 tablespoons unsweetened cocoa powder
- 1 to 2 teaspoons monk fruit extract or sugar-free sweetener
- ¼ teaspoon ground cinnamon
- ⅛ teaspoon salt
- Unsweetened whipped cream, for serving (optional)

1. In a microwave-safe mug or tall ramekin, combine the dark chocolate, butter, cream, and vanilla and microwave for 20 to 30 seconds. Remove and whisk to blend well.

2. Whisk in the cocoa powder, sweetener, cinnamon, and salt until smooth.

3. Microwave on high for 60 to 90 seconds, until set on top. The time will vary depending on the strength of the microwave.

4. Serve warm, directly out of the mug or invert the ramekin onto a plate and top with whipped cream (if using).

Per Serving: Calories: 352; Total Fat: 34g; Total Carbs: 15g; Net Carbs: 11g; Fiber: 4g; Protein: 7g; Sodium: 281mg; **Macros:** Fat: 87%, Carbs: 5%, Protein: 8%

AB AND J CHIA PUDDING

Serves 4 | Prep Time: 10 minutes, plus 6 hours to chill | Dairy-Free, Egg-Free, Gluten-Free, Vegetarian

With the nostalgic flavor of a peanut butter and jelly sandwich, this treat, high in omega-3 fatty acids, uses almond butter in place of the pro-inflammatory peanut butter and real fruit instead of sugar-laden jelly. Feel free to mix up the fruit flavors to create your own variations.

1 cup unsweetened almond milk
2 tablespoons unsweetened almond butter
½ cup fresh or frozen raspberries
1 teaspoon vanilla extract
1 to 2 teaspoons monk fruit extract (optional)
½ cup chia seeds

1. In a blender or tall narrow container (if using an immersion blender), combine the almond milk, almond butter, raspberries, vanilla, and monk fruit extract (if using) and blend until smooth.

2. Transfer the mixture to a medium bowl and add the chia seeds, whisking well to combine.

3. Divide the mixture between ramekins. Cover and refrigerate for at least 6 hours, preferably overnight. Serve cold.

Per Serving (½ cup): Calories: 188; Total Fat: 12g; Total Carbs: 14g; Net Carbs: 2g; Fiber: 12g; Protein: 6g; Sodium: 43mg;
Macros: Fat: 57%, Carbs: 30%, Protein: 13%

LEMON-BLUEBERRY ICE CREAM

Serves 8 | Prep Time: 10 minutes, plus 12 hours to freeze the bowl | Cook Time: 25 minutes, plus 6 hours to chill | Gluten-Free, Nut-Free, Vegetarian

This tastes like summer in a bowl. Many commercial keto-friendly ice creams are filled with sugar alcohols, which cause digestive distress, and other fillers, which can be very pro-inflammatory. This all-natural version leaves out all the junk.

- 1 cup fresh or thawed frozen blueberries
- Grated zest and juice of 1 lemon
- 1 to 2 teaspoons monk fruit extract
- ⅓ cup powdered sugar-free sweetener
- 2 large egg yolks
- 2 cups heavy whipping cream
- 1 teaspoon vanilla extract

1. Freeze the bowl of an ice cream maker for at least 12 hours or overnight.
2. In a medium bowl, combine the blueberries, lemon zest and juice, and monk fruit extract and mash well with the back of a fork. Alternatively, blend using an immersion blender for a smoother texture.
3. In a large bowl, whisk together the sweetener and egg yolks.
4. In a small saucepan, heat the cream over medium heat, until just below a boil. Remove from the heat and allow to cool slightly.
5. Slowly pour the warm cream into the egg yolk mixture, whisking constantly to avoid cooking the eggs. Return the eggs and cream to the saucepan over low heat.
6. Whisking constantly, cook for 15 to 20 minutes, until thickened. Remove from the heat and whisk in the blueberry mixture and vanilla. Transfer to a glass bowl and cool to room temperature. Cover and refrigerate for at least 6 hours.
7. Freeze the custard in an ice cream maker according to the manufacturer's directions. Serve.

VARIATION TIP: Feel free to mix up the flavor combination. I love strawberries with lime or blackberries with orange.

Per Serving (½ cup): Calories: 229; Total Fat: 23g; Total Carbs: 15g; Net Carbs: 14g; Fiber: 1g; Protein: 3g; Sodium: 18mg;
Macros: Fat: 90%, Carbs: 5%, Protein: 5%

CAULIFLOWER RICE PUDDING

Serves 4 | Prep Time: 5 minutes | Cook Time: 25 minutes, plus 4 hours to chill | Gluten-Free, Nut-Free, Vegetarian

When I was a child, my best friend's mom used to make her famous rice pudding, and we'd eat gobs of it during hours of long swim meets. This is a true comfort dessert for me. With all the cinnamon flavor and texture of the original recipe, I've created a keto-friendly version that brings me back in time and you won't even notice it's cauliflower and not rice!

1½ cups half-and-half
1 cinnamon stick
2 cups fresh riced cauliflower
4 large egg yolks
3 tablespoons monk fruit extract
1 teaspoon ground cinnamon

1. In a medium saucepan, combine the half-and-half and cinnamon stick and bring to just below a boil over medium-high heat, stirring occasionally.

2. Add the cauliflower, reduce the heat to low, and simmer for 8 minutes, until the liquid is mostly absorbed.

3. In a small bowl, beat the egg yolks. Add 1 tablespoon of cauliflower to the egg yolks and whisk for 30 seconds. Repeat this step two more times, whisking well after each 1-tablespoon addition. Then, add the monk fruit extract.

4. Add the egg yolk mixture to the saucepan and, whisking constantly, simmer for 5 minutes, or until thickened. Remove from the heat and cool to room temperature.

5. Remove the cinnamon stick and divide the mixture between small ramekins (or store the entire batch in a larger bowl) and top with the ground cinnamon. Refrigerate for at least 4 hours before serving cold.

Per Serving: Calories: 188; Total Fat: 15g; Total Carbs: 8g; Net Carbs: 7g; Fiber: 1g; Protein: 7g; Sodium: 73mg;
Macros: Fat: 72%, Carbs: 13%, Protein: 15%

MATCHA ICE CREAM

Serves 8 | Prep Time: 5 minutes, plus 12 hours to freeze the bowl | Cook Time: 25 minutes, plus 6 hours to freeze | Gluten-Free, Nut-Free, Vegetarian

Matcha is a powder made from high-quality whole green tea leaves, making it a very potent antioxidant and anti-inflammatory compound. Matcha ice cream and desserts are common in Japan and are gaining popularity worldwide.

1 tablespoon matcha green tea powder
½ teaspoon ground ginger
⅛ teaspoon freshly ground black pepper
4 large egg yolks
⅓ cup powdered sugar-free sweetener
2 cups half-and-half (or 1 cup heavy whipping cream and 1 cup whole milk)
1 teaspoon vanilla extract
¼ cup extra-virgin olive oil

1. Freeze the bowl of an ice cream maker for at least 12 hours or overnight.

2. In a small bowl, combine the matcha powder, ginger, and pepper. Set aside.

3. In a large bowl, whisk together the egg yolks and sweetener.

4. In a small saucepan, heat the half-and-half over medium heat until just below a boil. Remove from the heat and allow to cool slightly.

5. Slowly pour the warm half-and-half into the egg yolk mixture, whisking constantly to avoid cooking the eggs. Return the eggs and cream to the saucepan over low heat.

6. Whisking constantly, cook for 15 to 20 minutes, until thickened. Remove from the heat and whisk in the vanilla and matcha powder mixture. Whisking, stream in the olive oil until smooth and well combined. Transfer to a glass bowl and allow to cool to room temperature. Cover and refrigerate for at least 6 hours.

7. Freeze the custard in an ice cream maker according to the manufacturer's directions. Serve.

VARIATION TIP: If you don't have an ice cream maker, refrigerate for at least 12 hours. Whip the custard using an electric mixer until doubled in volume, and freeze before serving.

Per Serving (½ cup): Calories: 170; Total Fat: 16g; Total Carbs: 13g; Net Carbs: 13g; Fiber: 0g; Protein: 4g; Sodium: 41mg;
Macros: Fat: 85%, Carbs: 6%, Protein: 9%

COCONUT-ORANGE CUPCAKES

Makes 6 cupcakes | Prep Time: 15 minutes | Cook Time: 20 minutes | Dairy-Free, Gluten-Free, Vegetarian

Topped with a dollop of whipped cream, these have all the flavor of an orange creamsicle. Most gluten-free baked goods using almond flour contain xanthan gum for texture. I have found that smaller cakes baked in liners don't require the extra expensive ingredient. You can adjust the sweetener to your taste, but all the natural orange really imparts great flavor.

¼ cup powdered sugar-free sweetener
1 large egg
½ cup coconut oil, melted
1 teaspoon vanilla extract
½ cup coconut flour
½ cup almond flour
½ teaspoon baking powder
½ teaspoon salt
Grated zest and juice of 1 orange

1. Preheat the oven to 350°F and place liners into six cups of a muffin tin.

2. In a large bowl, whisk together the sweetener and egg. Add the coconut oil and vanilla and whisk until well combined.

3. In a medium bowl, whisk together the coconut flour, almond flour, baking powder, and salt. Add the dry ingredients and orange zest and juice to the wet ingredients and stir until just combined.

4. Divide the batter evenly among the prepared muffin tin and bake for 15 to 18 minutes, until a toothpick inserted in the center of a cupcake comes out clean.

5. Remove the cupcakes from the oven and cool for 5 minutes in the tin before transferring to a wire rack to cool completely.

Per Serving (1 cupcake): Calories: 277; Total Fat: 25g; Total Carbs: 19g; Net Carbs: 15g; Fiber: 4g; Protein: 4g; Sodium: 269mg; **Macros:** Fat: 81%, Carbs: 13%, Protein: 6%

CHAI TEA COOKIES

Makes 1 dozen cookies | Prep Time: 10 minutes | Cook Time: 20 minutes | Gluten-Free, Vegetarian

Chai is a traditional Indian beverage made by brewing black tea with fragrant anti-inflammatory spices and herbs, often combined with frothed milk or cream and sugar. These cookies have all the healing properties and unique flavor without all the pro-inflammatory sugars.

½ cup (1 stick) unsalted butter, at room temperature
⅓ cup granulated sugar-free sweetener
1 large egg
½ teaspoon vanilla extract
1 cup almond flour
1 cup coconut flour
½ teaspoon xanthan gum
½ teaspoon baking powder
½ teaspoon ground cinnamon
½ teaspoon ground cardamom
½ teaspoon ground ginger
½ teaspoon salt
¼ teaspoon freshly ground black pepper

1. Preheat the oven to 350°F. Line a baking sheet with parchment paper and set aside.

2. In a large bowl, using an electric mixer on medium speed, cream together the butter and sweetener until smooth. Add the egg and vanilla and beat well.

3. Add the almond and coconut flours, xanthan gum, baking powder, cinnamon, cardamom, ginger, salt, and pepper, and stir until well incorporated.

4. Using a spoon, place mounds of dough, about 1 inch in diameter, onto the prepared baking sheet about 1 inch apart.

5. Bake the cookies for 15 to 18 minutes, until set and lightly golden. Refrigerate for at least 1 hour before serving. Cookies can be stored in an airtight container at room temperature for two to three days or in the refrigerator for up to a week.

INGREDIENT TIP: You can increase the baking powder to 1 teaspoon and omit the xanthan gum, which tends to be pricey, but this will result in a crumblier cookie.

Per Serving (1 cookie): Calories: 170; Total Fat: 14g; Total Carbs: 13g; Net Carbs: 8g; Fiber: 5g; Protein: 4g; Sodium: 207mg;
Macros: Fat: 74%, Carbs: 17%, Protein: 9%

MATCHA FAT BOMBS

Makes 8 balls | **Prep Time:** 10 minutes, plus 1 hour 15 minutes to chill | Egg-Free, Gluten-Free, Vegetarian

Fat bombs are easy ways to get an extra dose of fat as part of a meal or as a satiating snack to keep ketogenic ratios on point. They are convenient and a little goes a long way, so they're great for road trips or busy workdays. This bomb has the added bonus of antioxidant-rich matcha for wonderful flavor and optimal nutrition.

- 8 ounces full-fat cream cheese, at room temperature
- ¼ cup almond flour
- 1 tablespoon matcha green tea powder
- 1 to 2 teaspoons monk fruit extract (optional)
- 1 teaspoon vanilla extract
- ½ teaspoon ground ginger
- ¼ cup finely chopped slivered almonds

1. In a mixing bowl, combine the cream cheese, almond flour, matcha, monk fruit extract (if using), vanilla, and ginger and stir well with a spatula. Place the bowl in the freezer for 15 minutes.

2. Using your hands, form the chilled mixture into eight (1-inch) balls.

3. Place the almonds in a shallow bowl. Roll the balls in the nuts to coat and place in the refrigerator to harden for at least 1 hour before serving. Store in an airtight container in the refrigerator for up to one week or in the freezer for up to two months.

INGREDIENT TIP: For a dairy-free version, substitute ½ cup cacao butter or coconut oil at room temperature for the cream cheese and chill an additional 15 minutes before forming into balls.

Per Serving (1 fat bomb): Calories: 146; Total Fat: 13g; Total Carbs: 4g; Net Carbs: 3g; Fiber: 1g; Protein: 4g; Sodium: 90mg; **Macros:** Fat: 80%, Carbs: 9%, Protein: 11%

SALTED MACADAMIA FAT BOMBS

Makes 8 balls | Prep Time: 10 minutes, plus 1 hour to chill | Dairy-Free, Egg-Free, Gluten-Free, Vegetarian

Aside from being quite delicious, macadamia nuts have the highest fat content of all nuts, making them very popular for ketogenic dieters. Consider this the ultimate fat bomb! If you can't find macadamia nut butter, you can grind your own using a food processor or substitute cashew butter here.

- ½ cup no-sugar-added macadamia nut butter
- ½ cup coconut oil
- ¼ cup coconut flour
- 1 to 2 teaspoons monk fruit extract (optional)
- 1½ teaspoons salt, divided
- ¼ cup finely chopped macadamia nuts

1. In a mixing bowl, combine the macadamia nut butter, coconut oil, coconut flour, monk fruit extract (if using), and ½ teaspoon of salt and stir well with a spatula to combine.

2. Using your hands, form the mixture into eight (1-inch) balls.

3. In a small bowl, combine the nuts and the remaining 1 teaspoon of salt. Roll the balls in the nuts and place in the refrigerator to harden for at least 1 hour before serving. Store in an airtight container in the refrigerator for up to one week or in the freezer for up to two months.

Per Serving (1 fat bomb): Calories: 254; Total Fat: 26g; Total Carbs: 7g; Net Carbs: 3g; Fiber: 4g; Protein: 1g; Sodium: 450mg; **Macros:** Fat: 92%, Carbs: 6%, Protein: 2%

LIME-COCONUT FAT BOMBS

Makes 8 balls | Prep Time: 10 minutes, plus 1 hour to chill | Dairy-Free, Egg-Free, Gluten-Free, Vegetarian

I love these stored in the freezer and enjoyed on a hot day. The mixture will be sticky until it hardens in the refrigerator or freezer and will become mushy if kept out for too long, so be sure to pack them with ice if you plan to travel with them.

½ cup coconut oil
½ cup coconut flour
½ cup unsweetened coconut flakes, divided
Grated zest and juice of 1 lime
1 to 2 teaspoons monk fruit extract (optional)
½ teaspoon salt

1. In a mixing bowl, combine the coconut oil, coconut flour, ¼ cup of coconut flakes, lime zest and juice, monk fruit extract (if using), and salt and stir well with a spatula to combine.

2. Using your hands, form the mixture into eight (1-inch) balls.

3. Place the remaining ¼ cup of coconut flakes in a shallow dish and roll the balls in it. Place the fat bombs in the refrigerator to harden for at least 1 hour before serving. Store in an airtight container in the refrigerator for up to one week or in the freezer for up to two months.

Per Serving (1 fat bomb): Calories: 186; Total Fat: 18g; Total Carbs: 6g; Net Carbs: 3g; Fiber: 3g; Protein: 1g; Sodium: 164mg; **Macros:** Fat: 87%, Carbs: 11%, Protein: 2%

COOKIE DOUGH FAT BOMBS

Makes 8 balls | Prep Time: 15 minutes, plus 2 hours to chill | Egg-Free, Gluten-Free, Vegetarian

Who doesn't love cookie dough? With this satiating fat bomb, now you can enjoy it without the guilt! These would also be delicious with the addition of chopped pecans or walnuts for nut lovers.

- ½ cup (1 stick) unsalted butter, at room temperature
- ¼ cup granulated sugar-free sweetener
- ½ teaspoon vanilla extract
- 1 cup almond flour
- ¼ cup coconut flour
- ½ teaspoon ground cinnamon
- ⅓ cup chopped dark chocolate (86 percent or higher) or sugar-free chocolate chips

1. In a large bowl, using an electric mixer on medium speed, cream together the butter and sweetener until smooth. Add the vanilla and beat well.
2. Add the almond flour, coconut flour, and cinnamon and stir until well incorporated. Stir in the chopped chocolate and mix well.
3. Using a spoon or your hands, form the mixture into eight (1-inch) balls and place on a baking sheet lined with parchment paper. Refrigerate for at least 2 hours before serving. Store in an airtight container in the refrigerator for up to one week or in the freezer for up to two months.

Per Serving (1 fat bomb): Calories: 163; Total Fat: 15g; Total Carbs: 12g; Net Carbs: 10g; Fiber: 2g; Protein: 1g; Sodium: 100mg; **Macros:** Fat: 83%, Carbs: 15%, Protein: 2%

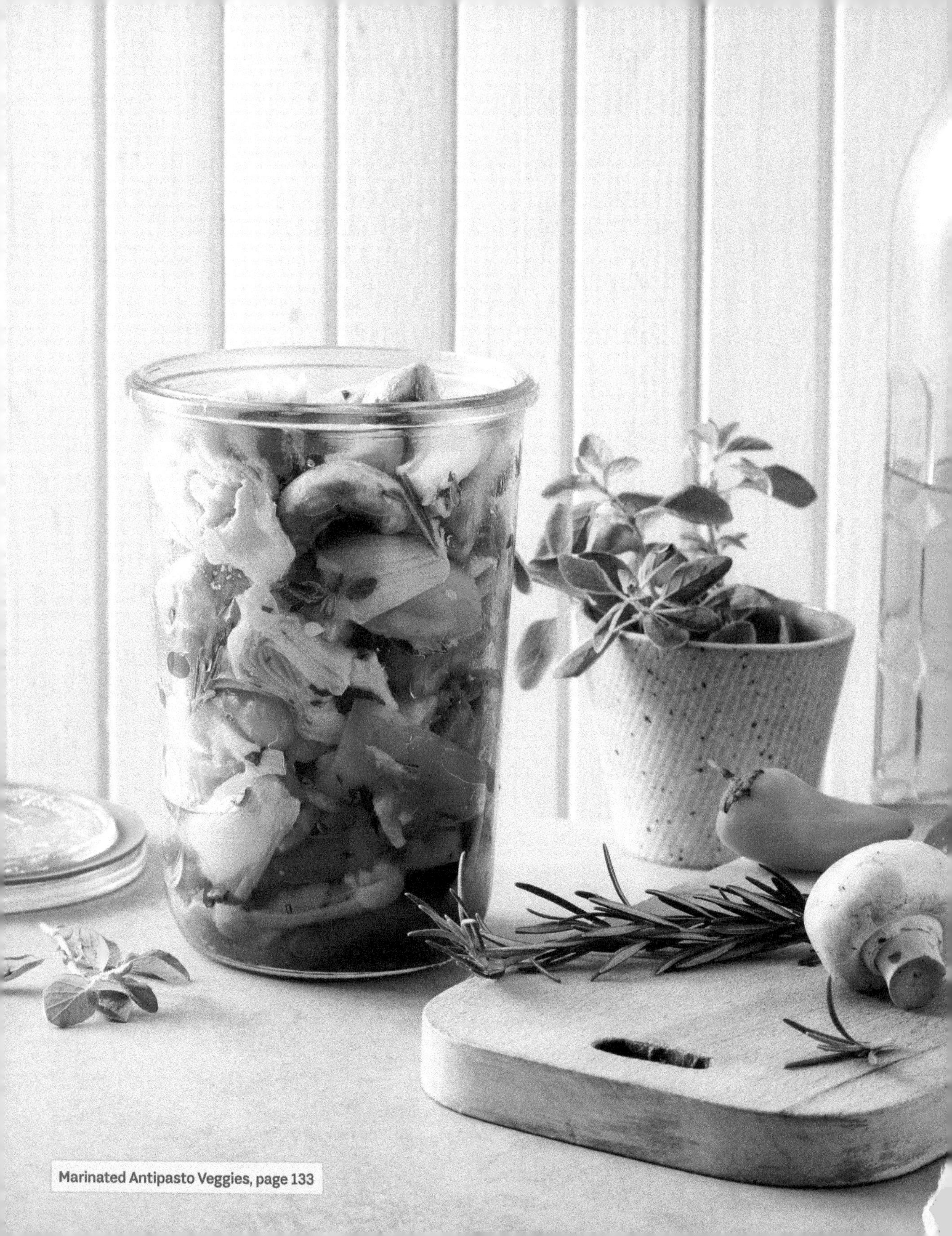

Marinated Antipasto Veggies, page 133

CHAPTER NINE

Snacks and Small Bites

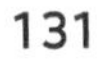

ANTI-INFLAMMATORY POWER BITES

Makes 1 dozen bites | Prep Time: 20 minutes, plus 1 hour to chill | Dairy-Free, Egg-Free, Gluten-Free, Vegetarian

These are a staple in our house for an on-the-go snack. So many manufactured "bar" products are full of sugars and other fillers and those that are "low carb" usually contain artificial sweeteners or sugar alcohols, which can disrupt gut health. These are simple to make and can be amended to fit your preferences. Simply choose the type of seed or nut butter you desire.

- 1 cup unsweetened almond butter
- ½ cup ground flaxseed
- ¼ cup almond or coconut flour
- ¼ cup unsweetened cocoa powder
- ¼ cup unsweetened coconut flakes
- ¼ cup roasted pumpkin seeds
- ¼ cup chia seeds
- 1 teaspoon ground cinnamon
- 1 to 2 teaspoons monk fruit extract (optional)

1. In a large bowl, combine the almond butter, flaxseed, almond flour, cocoa powder, coconut flakes, pumpkin seeds, chia seeds, cinnamon, and monk fruit extract (if using).

2. Using your hands, mix everything together and shape the mixture into 12 (1-inch) balls. Place them in a single layer on a baking sheet or in a large container. Cover and refrigerate for at least 1 hour before serving.

3. Store the balls in an airtight container in the refrigerator for up to one week or in the freezer for up to three months.

INGREDIENT TIP: Natural nut butters, such as almond, do not contain processed oils like palm oil. The natural almond oil will rise to the top. Be sure to stir the almond butter very well before using to prevent these from being too runny. For best results, use almond butter that has been refrigerated for at least 12 hours and use when cold.

Per Serving (1 bite): Calories: 214; Total Fat: 18g; Total Carbs: 9g; Net Carbs: 3g; Fiber: 6g; Protein: 8g; Sodium: 10mg;
Macros: Fat: 76%, Carbs: 9%, Protein: 15%

MARINATED ANTIPASTO VEGGIES

Serves 8 | Prep Time: 10 minutes, plus 24 hours to marinate | Dairy-Free, Egg-Free, Gluten-Free, Nut-Free, Vegetarian

Antipasto is traditionally served before the main course of many Italian meals. These antipasto veggies are perfect to store in the refrigerator for a quick and easy snack or as part of an appetizer spread to wow guests.

- 1 (14-ounce) can artichoke hearts, drained and quartered
- 1 cup halved small button mushrooms
- 8 small snack-size sweet peppers, seeded and halved, or 2 bell peppers, cut into 1-inch-thick strips
- ¾ cup extra-virgin olive oil
- 4 small garlic cloves, peeled and crushed
- 1 tablespoon chopped fresh rosemary
- 1 tablespoon chopped fresh oregano, or 1 teaspoon dried oregano
- 1 to 2 teaspoons red pepper flakes
- 1 teaspoon salt

1. In a medium bowl, combine the artichoke hearts, mushrooms, peppers, olive oil, garlic, rosemary, oregano, red pepper flakes, and salt. Toss to combine well.

2. Place the mixture in an airtight glass container in the refrigerator to marinate for at least 24 hours before serving. The marinated veggies can be stored in the refrigerator for up to two weeks.

VARIATION TIP: These marinated vegetables are delicious tossed with zucchini noodles for a quick and easy vegetarian meal. Top with leftover grilled chicken, meat, or fish to add protein.

Per Serving: Calories: 218; Total Fat: 22g; Total Carbs: 5g; Net Carbs: 3g; Fiber: 2g; Protein: 1g; Sodium: 404mg; **Macros:** Fat: 91%; Carbs: 7%, Protein: 2%

CRAB AND ARTICHOKE DIP

Makes 2 cups | Prep Time: 10 minutes | Cook Time: 25 minutes | Gluten-Free, Nut-Free

Loaded with veggies for added nutrition, this dip is a crowd-pleaser. I serve it with an array of crunchy raw vegetables, such as celery, cucumber rounds, or sliced peppers, and I mix the leftovers into scrambled eggs the next morning. You can omit the crab if desired; simply increase the spinach by ½ cup.

- 2 tablespoons extra-virgin olive oil
- ½ small onion, chopped
- ½ cup chopped artichoke hearts
- 1 cup frozen spinach, thawed and drained
- 2 garlic cloves, minced
- 8 ounces full-fat cream cheese, at room temperature
- 4 ounces crab meat
- 1 teaspoon smoked paprika
- 1 teaspoon salt or Old Bay seasoning
- ½ to 1 teaspoon red pepper flakes
- ¼ cup Anti-Inflammatory Mayo (page 148)
- ¼ cup freshly shredded Parmesan cheese

1. Preheat the oven to 375°F.

2. In a medium skillet, heat the olive oil over medium heat. Add the onion and sauté for 6 minutes, until it is tender. Add the artichokes and spinach and sauté for 4 to 5 minutes, or until the vegetables are tender and any water has evaporated.

3. Add the garlic and cream cheese and, stirring constantly, cook for 3 to 4 minutes, until the cheese is melted and creamy.

4. Reduce the heat to low and stir in the crab meat, paprika, salt, and red pepper flakes. Remove from the heat and stir in the mayo until creamy and well combined.

5. Transfer the mixture to an 8-inch-square glass baking dish, spreading it out evenly. Top with the Parmesan and bake for 8 to 10 minutes, until the cheese is melted and lightly browned. Serve warm.

MAKE AHEAD: The mixture can be made ahead and stored covered in the refrigerator for up to four days, before baking and serving.

Per Serving (⅓ cup): Calories: 308; Total Fat: 29g; Total Carbs: 6g; Net Carbs: 5g; Fiber: 1g; Protein: 8g; Sodium: 758mg;
Macros: Fat: 85%, Carbs: 5%, Protein: 10%

LOADED FETA

Makes 1½ cups | Prep Time: 5 minutes | Egg-Free, Gluten-Free, Nut-Free, Vegetarian

Cheese is a favorite keto-friendly snack, but as it is often high in protein, too much can knock macronutrient ratios off. Pairing cheeses with fats, such as the oil in this recipe, helps keep portions in check and macros in line.

⅓ cup extra-virgin olive oil
2 teaspoons dried rosemary
1 teaspoon dried oregano
1 teaspoon dried thyme
1 to 2 teaspoons red pepper flakes
½ teaspoon salt
8 ounces sheep's milk feta cheese, cut into ½-inch cubes

1. In a medium bowl or large glass jar, whisk together the olive oil, rosemary, oregano, thyme, red pepper flakes, and salt. Add the feta and toss to coat, being sure not to crumble the feta.

2. Store, covered, in the refrigerator for up to four days. Let sit at room temperature for at least 30 minutes before serving to allow the oil to return to liquid.

VARIATION TIP: You can make this into more of a dip or spread by mashing the feta until crumbled and mixed well with the oil.

Per Serving (⅓ cup): Calories: 311; Total Fat: 30g; Total Carbs: 3g; Net Carbs: 2g; Fiber: 1g; Protein: 8g; Sodium: 941mg;
Macros: Fat: 87%, Carbs: 3%, Protein: 10%

HERBY YOGURT DIP

Makes about 1½ cups | Prep Time: 10 minutes | Egg-Free, Gluten-Free, Nut-Free, Vegetarian

This dip is great paired with raw veggies for a snack, but you can mix it into tuna or chicken salad for a unique flavor twist. Or pair it with simple grilled meats or fish to add flavor and healthy fat to the meal.

1 cup plain whole milk Greek yogurt
¼ cup extra-virgin olive oil
¼ cup chopped fresh parsley
1 tablespoon freshly squeezed lemon juice
1 tablespoon chopped fresh dill, or 1 teaspoon dried dill
1 tablespoon chopped fresh oregano, or 1 teaspoon dried oregano
1 teaspoon garlic powder
1 teaspoon salt
½ teaspoon freshly ground black pepper
Assorted raw vegetables, for serving

1. In a medium bowl, combine the yogurt, olive oil, parsley, lemon juice, dill, oregano, garlic powder, salt, and pepper and whisk well until smooth and creamy.

2. Serve with raw vegetables. Store the dip in an airtight container in the refrigerator for up to four days.

VARIATION TIP: Add an additional ¼ cup of olive oil to make a thinner dressing for salads or grilled vegetables.

Per Serving (¼ cup): Calories: 118; Total Fat: 11g; Total Carbs: 2g; Net Carbs: 2g; Fiber: <1g; Protein: 4g; Sodium: 410mg; **Macros:** Fat: 84%, Carbs: 2%, Protein: 14%

SMOKED SALMON AND GOAT CHEESE PINWHEELS

Serves 4 | Prep Time: 15 minutes | Egg-Free, Gluten-Free, Nut-Free

Smoked salmon and goat cheese make one of my favorite flavor combinations, and this impressive snack comes together in a flash. Serve with mixed greens tossed with Basic Vinaigrette (page 147), and these can easily become a light meal.

4 ounces goat cheese
¼ cup extra-virgin olive oil, divided
1 tablespoon finely chopped capers
1 tablespoon minced red onion
1 teaspoon dried dill
¼ to ½ teaspoon red pepper flakes
6 ounces smoked wild-caught salmon (not cut nova bits), thinly sliced into 2 rough rectangles

1. In a small bowl, mix together the goat cheese, 2 tablespoons of olive oil, capers, onion, dill, and red pepper flakes.

2. Lay out the slices of smoked salmon on a large plate or serving dish. Top each slice with the goat cheese mixture and spread to evenly coat. Starting at the narrow end, roll each slice of salmon to form a log. Slice each log into 1-inch segments and arrange on the platter.

3. Drizzle the pinwheels with the remaining 2 tablespoons of olive oil and serve chilled.

VARIATION TIP: You can substitute cream cheese for the goat cheese if preferred.

Per Serving: Calories: 274; Total Fat: 24g; Total Carbs: 1g; Net Carbs: 1g; Fiber: <1g; Protein: 14g; Sodium: 455mg; **Macros:** Fat: 79%, Carbs: 1%, Protein: 20%

SALMON SALAD SUSHI BITES

Serves 4 to 6 | Prep Time: 20 minutes | Dairy-Free, Gluten-Free, Nut-Free

These pretty bite-size snacks are fancy enough to serve at a cocktail party and fun enough to stick into your kids' lunchboxes! This recipe calls for canned salmon for convenience and budget, but feel free to substitute fresh or smoked salmon if you prefer the flavor. Look for nori in the Asian section of your grocery store or in Asian markets.

2 large cucumbers, peeled
8 ounces canned red salmon, preferably sockeye, bones and skin removed
¼ cup Anti-Inflammatory Mayo (page 148)
1 tablespoon sesame oil
2 teaspoons miso paste
1 teaspoon sriracha or other hot sauce
1 nori seaweed sheet, crumbled
½ avocado, thinly sliced

1. Slice the cucumber into 1-inch segments and, using a spoon, scrape the seeds out of the center of each segment and place center-side up on a plate.

2. In a medium bowl, combine the salmon, mayo, sesame oil, miso, sriracha, and nori and mix until creamy.

3. Spoon the salmon mixture into the center of each cucumber segment and top with a slice of avocado. Serve chilled.

MAKE AHEAD: The salmon salad mixture can be made up to 24 hours in advance and stored in an airtight container in the refrigerator until you are ready to stuff the cucumbers.

Per Serving (2 pieces): Calories: 289; Total Fat: 24g; Total Carbs: 8g; Net Carbs: 5g; Fiber: 3g; Protein: 13g; Sodium: 373mg;
Macros: Fat: 75%, Carbs: 7%, Protein: 18%

SEEDY CRACKERS

Serves 4 | Prep Time: 20 minutes | Cook Time: 15 minutes | Dairy-Free, Gluten-Free, Vegetarian

For when you just need a crunch, these crackers are high in anti-inflammatory fats and herbs and very low in carbohydrates. Enjoy them paired with a higher-fat topping such as Spiced Guacamole (page 152) or Olive and Artichoke Tapenade (page 154) to keep the macronutrient ratios keto-friendly.

1 cup almond flour
1 tablespoon sesame seeds
1 tablespoon flaxseed
1 tablespoon fennel seed
¼ teaspoon baking soda
¼ teaspoon salt
Freshly ground black pepper
1 large egg, at room temperature
1 tablespoon extra-virgin olive oil

1. Preheat the oven to 350°F. Line a baking sheet with parchment paper and set aside.

2. In a large bowl, combine the almond flour, sesame seeds, flaxseed, fennel seed, baking soda, salt, and pepper and stir well.

3. In a small bowl, whisk the egg until well beaten. Add the egg and olive oil to the dry ingredients and stir well to combine and form the dough into a ball.

4. Place one layer of parchment paper on the countertop and place the dough on top. Cover with a second layer of parchment and, using a rolling pin, roll the dough to ⅛-inch thickness, aiming for a rectangular shape.

5. Cut the dough into 1- to 2-inch crackers, transfer the crackers to the prepared baking sheet, and bake for 10 to 15 minutes, until crispy and slightly golden. Alternatively, bake the rolled dough prior to cutting and break into "free form" crackers once baked and crispy.

6. Store in an airtight container in the refrigerator for up to four days or the freezer for up to one month. Bring to room temperature before serving.

Per Serving: Calories: 238; Total Fat: 21g; Total Carbs: 7g; Net Carbs: 3g; Fiber: 4g; Protein: 9g; Sodium: 247mg;
Macros: Fat: 79%, Carbs: 6%, Protein: 15%

GOAT CHEESE CAPRESE SALAD

Serves 4 | Prep Time: 10 minutes | Egg-Free, Gluten-Free, Nut-Free, Vegetarian

The wonderful summery combination of vine ripe fresh tomatoes, fresh mozzarella, and basil stems from the island of Capri in Italy, giving this salad its name. In this version, perfect for a hearty snack, I substitute goat cheese for the traditional mozzarella for those who are sensitive to cow's milk. Feel free to use traditional fresh mozzarella if you prefer.

1 large ripe tomato
1 teaspoon salt, divided
1 (4-ounce) goat cheese log, cut into 4 equal pieces
8 whole fresh basil leaves, thinly sliced
¼ cup extra-virgin olive oil
1 tablespoon balsamic vinegar
½ teaspoon freshly ground black pepper

1. Slice the tomato into four thick slices and place them in a single layer on a plate or serving dish. Sprinkle with ½ teaspoon of salt.

2. Place a slice of goat cheese on each tomato slice and, using a knife, spread to cover the tomato. Top each with basil and drizzle each with 1 tablespoon of olive oil and ¼ tablespoon of vinegar.

3. Season with the remaining ½ teaspoon of salt and the pepper. Serve immediately.

Per Serving: Calories: 212; Total Fat: 21g; Total Carbs: 4g; Net Carbs: 3g; Fiber: 1g; Protein: 6g; Sodium: 704mg;
Macros: Fat: 84%, Carbs: 6%, Protein: 10%

PIMENTO CHEESE

Serves 4 to 6 | Prep Time: 5 minutes | Gluten-Free, Nut-Free, Vegetarian

Being from the South, I don't know many people who don't love this tangy, creamy goodness. A long-time client turned dear friend of mine shared her secret for perfect pimento cheese: adding cream cheese! The amazing result is delicious on its own, paired with Seedy Crackers (page 139) or celery sticks, or melted inside a Keto Sandwich Round (page 146) for the ultimate grilled cheese.

- 4 ounces full-fat cream cheese, at room temperature
- ¼ cup Anti-Inflammatory Mayo (page 148)
- 2 tablespoons pimentos, drained and chopped
- ½ teaspoon salt
- ¼ to ½ teaspoon cayenne pepper or red pepper flakes
- 1 cup freshly shredded extra-sharp Cheddar cheese

1. In a medium bowl, combine the cream cheese, mayo, pimentos, salt, and cayenne and whisk until well combined, smooth, and creamy. Stir in the Cheddar and mix until well incorporated.

2. Serve chilled or store covered in the refrigerator for up to four days.

INGREDIENT TIP: Most pimentos come in 2- to 4-ounce jars, so you will have leftovers if you don't double this recipe. They will last in the refrigerator for up to one week, but be sure to transfer them from the metal jar they come in to a sealed glass jar for best results. Chopped leftover pimentos are delicious added to green salads or mixed into an egg, tuna, or chicken salad.

Per Serving (2 tablespoons): Calories: 340; Total Fat: 33g; Total Carbs: 3g; Net Carbs: 3g; Fiber: <1g; Protein: 9g; Sodium: 647mg; **Macros:** Fat: 87%, Carbs: 2%, Protein: 11%

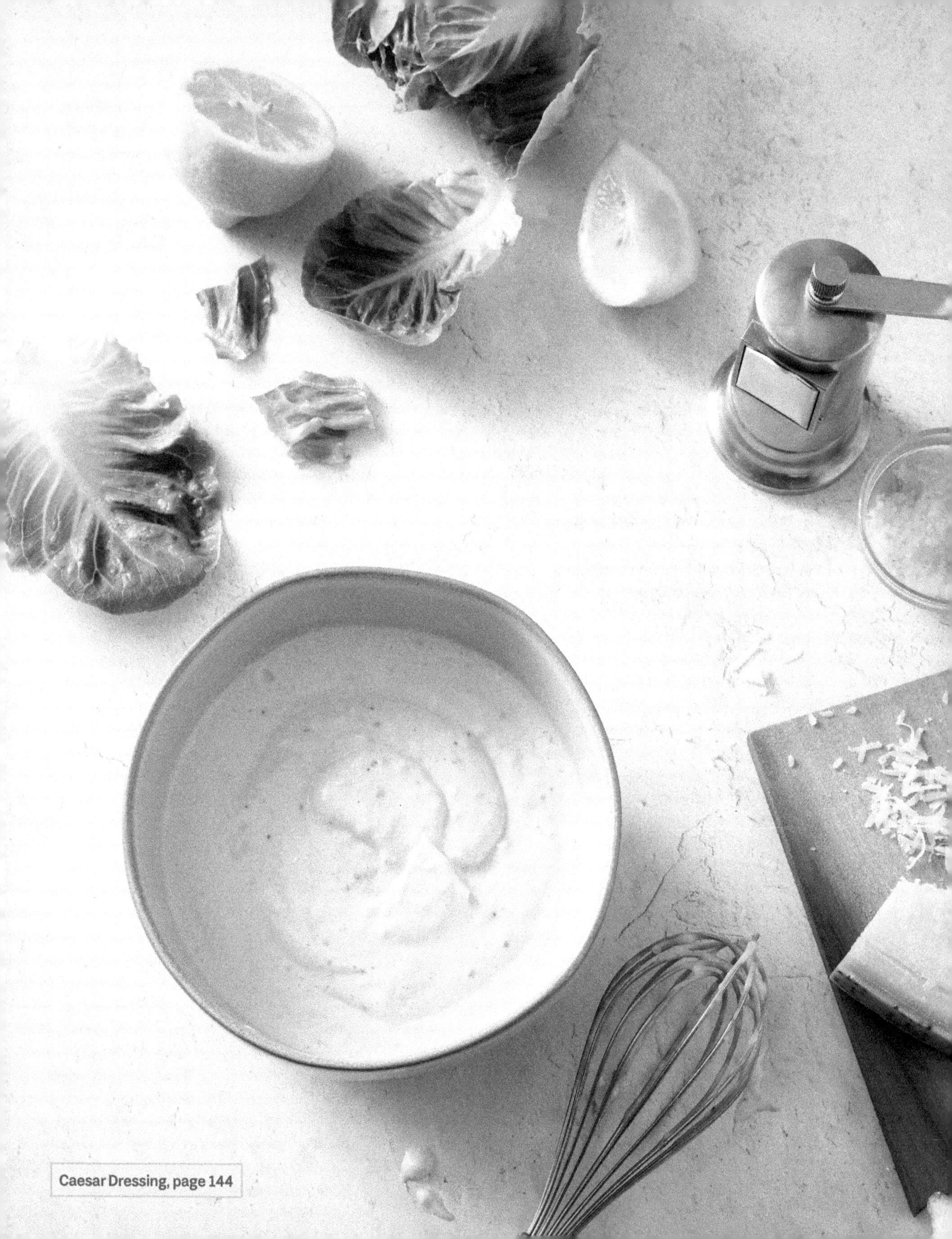

Caesar Dressing, page 144

CHAPTER TEN

Sauces and Staples

CAESAR DRESSING

Makes about 1½ cups | Prep Time: 10 minutes | Gluten-Free, Nut-Free

This is the only dressing my son will eat; it's that good! Even if you have an aversion to fish, don't omit the anchovy paste, as it is imperative to the wonderful flavor profile and adds a big bonus of anti-inflammatory omega-3 fatty acids. Delicious on any salad, it is especially wonderful tossed with crispy romaine lettuce and topped with a nice piece of grilled salmon and chunks of ripe avocado.

2 tablespoons freshly squeezed lemon juice
2 small garlic cloves, minced
1 teaspoon anchovy paste
1 teaspoon Dijon mustard
1 teaspoon Worcestershire sauce
1 cup Anti-Inflammatory Mayo (page 148)
½ cup freshly grated Parmesan cheese
¼ teaspoon salt
¼ teaspoon freshly ground black pepper

1. In a medium bowl, whisk together the lemon juice, garlic, anchovy paste, mustard, and Worcestershire sauce. Add the mayo, Parmesan, salt, and pepper and whisk until well combined. Taste and adjust the seasoning to your liking.

2. Store in an airtight container in the refrigerator for up to one week.

Per Serving (2 tablespoons): Calories: 189; Total Fat: 20g; Total Carbs: 1g; Net Carbs: 1g; Fiber: <1g; Protein: 2g; Sodium: 256mg; **Macros:** Fat: 95%, Carbs: 1%, Protein: 4%

GARLIC-BASIL ALFREDO SAUCE

Makes about 2 cups | Prep Time: 5 minutes | Cook Time: 10 minutes | Egg-Free, Gluten-Free, Nut-Free, Vegetarian

This rich and creamy sauce is wonderful tossed with zoodles or broccoli. Add chicken or shrimp for a heartier meal. This also serves as a wonderful base for a baked cauliflower casserole. The garlic and basil add wonderful flavor and anti-inflammatory properties.

- ½ cup (1 stick) unsalted butter
- 4 garlic cloves, minced
- 1 cup heavy whipping cream
- 4 ounces full-fat cream cheese
- 1½ cups freshly shredded Parmesan cheese
- 1 teaspoon salt
- 1 teaspoon freshly ground black pepper
- ⅓ cup chopped fresh basil

1. In a medium saucepan, melt the butter over medium-low heat, being careful not to burn it. Add the garlic and sauté for 2 minutes, or until fragrant.

2. Add the cream and cream cheese and whisk until melted and smooth. Whisk in the Parmesan, salt, and pepper and reduce the heat to low. Whisking constantly, cook for 3 to 4 minutes, until well combined and creamy.

3. Stir in the basil and serve warm.

Per Serving (⅓ cup): Calories: 452; Total Fat: 43g; Total Carbs: 4g; Net Carbs: 4g; Fiber: <1g; Protein: 13g; Sodium: 917mg; **Macros**: Fat: 86%, Carbs: 2%, Protein: 12%

KETO SANDWICH ROUND

Serves 1 | Prep Time: 5 minutes | Cook Time: 90 seconds | Dairy-Free, Gluten-Free, Vegetarian

So many commercial keto-friendly breads or wraps are filled with additives, artificial sweeteners, and other pro-inflammatory ingredients. Skip the slicing and serve this as a dinner roll or pull-apart bread option, or very thinly slice it into quarters, bake in the oven, and serve as a toast point with cheese or spreads. These don't store well, so I recommend only making what you plan on consuming in the moment.

3 tablespoons almond flour
1 large egg
1 tablespoon extra-virgin olive oil
1 teaspoon everything bagel seasoning (or ½ teaspoon salt and ½ teaspoon garlic powder)
¼ teaspoon baking powder

1. In a microwave-safe 4- to 5-inch ramekin or small bowl, combine the almond flour, egg, olive oil, everything seasoning, and baking powder. Mix well with a fork.

2. Microwave on high for 90 seconds.

3. Slide a knife around the edges of the ramekin and flip to remove the bread.

4. Slice the round in half with a serrated knife to make two pieces for a sandwich.

Per Serving: Calories: 338; Total Fat: 29g; Total Carbs: 5g; Net Carbs: 3g; Fiber: 2g; Protein: 11g; Sodium: 506mg; **Macros:** Fat: 77%, Carbs: 10%, Protein: 13%

BASIC VINAIGRETTE

Makes about ¾ cup | Prep Time: 5 minutes | Dairy-Free, Egg-Free, Gluten-Free, Nut-Free, Vegetarian

Most store-bought dressings, especially vinaigrettes, contain sugar and pro-inflammatory oils, such as canola or soybean oil. Making your own vinaigrette using anti-inflammatory oils is really quite simple and allows for variety, since you can use different herbs and spices.

- ½ cup avocado or extra-virgin olive oil
- ¼ cup white or red wine vinegar
- 1 tablespoon Dijon mustard
- 1 small garlic clove, pressed or minced (optional)
- 1 to 2 teaspoons dried rosemary, basil, parsley, thyme, or oregano
- ½ teaspoon salt
- ½ to 1 teaspoon red pepper flakes

1. In a glass jar with a lid, combine the avocado oil, vinegar, mustard, garlic (if using), rosemary, salt, and red pepper flakes and shake until well combined.

2. Store, covered, in the refrigerator for up to two weeks. Bring to room temperature and shake well before serving, as the oil and vinegar will naturally separate.

INGREDIENT TIP: A vinaigrette is just a combination of an oil and an acid (vinegar). You can use fresh lemon juice in place of the vinegar for a refreshing taste or a combination of the two.

Per Serving (2 tablespoons): Calories: 164; Total Fat: 18g; Total Carbs: <1g; Net Carbs: <1g; Fiber: <1g; Protein: <1g; Sodium: 257mg; **Macros:** Fat: 99%, Carbs: <1%, Protein: <1%

ANTI-INFLAMMATORY MAYO

Makes about 1 cup | Prep Time: 5 minutes | Dairy-Free, Gluten-Free, Nut-Free, Vegetarian

Most commercial mayonnaises are made with either canola or soybean oil, making them pro-inflammatory. Avocado oil–based mayonnaises are available, but they are very pricey. Once you get the hang of it, homemade healthy mayonnaise is a breeze to make and can save you a lot of money. Olive oil has a much less neutral flavor than avocado oil, and therefore is not used in this recipe, though it certainly can be if you prefer.

- 1 large egg, at room temperature
- 2 teaspoons white wine vinegar
- ½ to 1 teaspoon salt
- ¼ to ½ teaspoon ground turmeric
- 1 cup avocado oil

1. Crack the egg into the bottom of a wide-mouth jar. Carefully add the vinegar, salt, and turmeric.
2. Gently add the oil, being careful not to disturb the egg.
3. Carefully insert the immersion blender into the jar, allowing the blade casing to fully touch the bottom of the jar and sit flat. Blend on low for 25 to 30 seconds without moving the blender, until the egg begins to emulsify and the mixture starts to turn white and creamy. Continuing to blend on low, slowly move the blender toward the top of the jar, but remaining in the mixture. Move the blender up and down several times until the mayo is smooth and creamy.
4. Store, covered, in the refrigerator for up to two weeks.

INGREDIENT TIP: Making sure your egg is room temperature and not fresh out of the refrigerator is key to preventing a failed "broken" mayo. However, sometimes the egg does not want to emulsify, and the result is a chunky mess that just won't blend. Starting over is your best bet, but you can try to save it with the following method. Whisk a room temperature egg yolk in a small bowl. Add 1 tablespoon "broken" mayo and whisk vigorously until creamy. Continue with the remaining mayo until well blended and smooth.

Per Serving (1 tablespoon): Calories: 125; Total Fat: 14g; Total Carbs: <1g; Net Carbs: <1g; Fiber: 0g; Protein: <1g; Sodium: 78mg; **Macros:** Fat: 100%, Carbs: <1%, Protein: <1%

LEMON-TURMERIC AIOLI

Makes 1 cup | **Prep Time:** 5 minutes | Dairy-Free, Gluten-Free, Nut-Free, Vegetarian

An aioli is a thinner version of mayonnaise, but with added flavor from garlic and other herbs or spices. I find aioli to be a great way to add extra fat to simple meals of roasted or grilled proteins and veggies. Since turmeric can have a bitter taste, I balance this out with the addition of monk fruit extract. Feel free to omit this if you are a seasoned turmeric eater!

- 1 cup Anti-Inflammatory Mayo (page 148)
- Grated zest and juice of 1 lemon
- 2 garlic cloves, minced
- 1 teaspoon monk fruit extract (optional)
- 1 teaspoon ground turmeric
- ½ teaspoon cayenne pepper or red pepper flakes (optional)

1. In a small bowl, combine the mayo, lemon zest and juice, garlic, monk fruit extract (if using), turmeric, and cayenne (if using) and whisk until smooth and creamy.

2. Store the aioli, covered, in the refrigerator for up to one week.

VARIATION TIP: You can change the flavor profile by using different citrus (try orange or lime), spices, and/or herbs.

Per Serving (2 tablespoons): Calories: 254; Total Fat: 28g; Total Carbs: 1g; Net Carbs: 1g; Fiber: <1g; Protein: 1g; Sodium: 155mg; **Macros:** Fat: 99%, Carbs: <1%, Protein: <1%

GARLIC-ROSEMARY BUTTER

Makes ½ cup | Prep Time: 10 minutes | Egg-Free, Gluten-Free, Nut-Free, Vegetarian

One of the biggest struggles for new keto dieters is getting the right balance of fats at each meal. This flavored butter makes adding extra fats to grilled meats or fish and veggies tasty and full of variety.

½ cup (1 stick) unsalted butter, at room temperature
1 tablespoon finely chopped fresh rosemary, or 1 teaspoon dried rosemary
2 garlic cloves, minced
½ teaspoon salt

1. In a medium bowl, using an electric mixer on medium or using an immersion blender, blend the butter, rosemary, garlic, and salt until smooth and creamy.

2. Using a spatula, transfer the butter mixture to a small glass container and cover. Store in the refrigerator for up to one month or in the freezer for up to four months.

VARIATION TIP: You can change the flavor by changing up the herbs used. I love the combination of garlic and rosemary, but tarragon, oregano, and sage are also lovely.

Per Serving (1 tablespoon): Calories: 103; Total Fat: 12g; Total Carbs: <1g; Net Carbs: <1g; Fiber: <1g; Protein: <1g; Sodium: 239mg; **Macros:** Fat: 100%, Carbs: <1%, Protein: <1%

BASIL PESTO

Makes about 1 cup | Prep Time: 10 minutes | Egg-Free, Gluten-Free, Vegetarian

This condiment, packed with flavorful nutrition, is another versatile way to get extra fat into your diet without getting bored of the same flavors. So many store-bought versions use canola or other pro-inflammatory oils, so making your own is your best bet for fresh flavor and optimal nutrition.

- 4 cups packed whole fresh basil leaves
- ½ cup freshly shredded Parmesan cheese
- ¼ cup pine nuts
- 2 garlic cloves, peeled
- 1 teaspoon salt
- ½ teaspoon freshly ground black pepper
- ½ cup extra-virgin olive oil
- 1 tablespoon freshly squeezed lemon juice

1. In a food processor, combine the basil, Parmesan, pine nuts, and garlic and blend until very finely chopped. Add the salt and pepper.
2. With the processor running, stream in the olive oil and lemon juice until well blended. If the mixture seems too thick, add warm water, 1 tablespoon at a time, until the texture is smooth and creamy.
3. Store the pesto in an airtight container in the refrigerator for up to one week.

VARIATION TIP: Feel free to substitute other herbs or greens, such as parsley or arugula, for some or all of the basil. You can also opt for another nut, such as walnut or cashew, if you prefer.

Per Serving (2 tablespoons): Calories: 180; Total Fat: 18g; Total Carbs: 2g; Net Carbs: 1g; Fiber: 1g; Protein: 4g; Sodium: 382mg; **Macros:** Fat: 90%, Carbs: 1%, Protein: 9%

SPICED GUACAMOLE

Makes about 1½ cups | Prep Time: 10 minutes | Dairy-Free, Egg-Free, Gluten-Free, Nut-Free, Vegetarian

I could eat guacamole with everything! This version takes the traditional to a new level by adding extra anti-inflammatory power from olive oil and turmeric. I love a chunky guac, but if you prefer yours to be creamier, you can pass it through a food processor or immersion blender to create a more consistent texture.

- 2 very ripe avocados, pitted and peeled, pits reserved
- Juice of ½ lemon
- 2 tablespoons extra-virgin olive oil
- 1 garlic clove, pressed or minced
- 1 tablespoon minced red onion
- 1 tablespoon chopped jalapeño (optional)
- 1 teaspoon salt
- ½ to 1 teaspoon ground turmeric
- ½ teaspoon freshly ground black pepper
- ¼ to ½ cup chopped fresh cilantro (optional)

In a medium bowl, combine the avocados, lemon juice, olive oil, and garlic and mash well with a fork. Stir in the onion, jalapeño (if using), salt, turmeric, pepper, and cilantro (if using) until well combined. Serve immediately.

COOKING TIP: To store leftover guacamole and minimize browning, place the two reserved pits in the guacamole and cover completely with plastic wrap, pushing the plastic to touch the surface and prevent any oxygen from reaching the guacamole.

Per Serving (⅓ cup): Calories: 157; Total Fat: 15g; Total Carbs: 6g; Net Carbs: 2g; Fiber: 4g; Protein: 1g; Sodium: 524mg; **Macros:** Fat: 86%, Carbs: 11%, Protein: 3%

EASY MARINARA SAUCE

Makes 8 cups | Prep Time: 15 minutes | Cook Time: 1 hour | Egg-Free, Gluten-Free, Nut-Free, Vegetarian

Most store-bought marinara sauces are loaded with added sugars and lack the healthy fats of olive oil. This version is full of flavor and is a breeze to make. Most of the cooking time is inactive and the longer the sauce simmers, the deeper the flavor. Even if you are in a weeknight rush, this can come together in as little as 30 minutes.

- ½ cup extra-virgin olive oil, divided
- 2 tablespoons unsalted butter
- 1 red bell pepper, minced
- ½ small onion, minced
- 4 garlic cloves, minced
- 2 (32-ounce) cans crushed tomatoes
- 2 tablespoons chopped fresh oregano, or 1 teaspoon dried oregano
- 2 teaspoons salt
- ½ to 1 teaspoon red pepper flakes
- ½ cup chopped fresh basil

1. In a large skillet, heat 2 tablespoons of olive oil and the butter over medium-low heat. Cook the bell pepper and onion for about 5 minutes, until just tender. Add the garlic and sauté for 2 minutes, or until fragrant.

2. Stir in the tomatoes and their juices, oregano, salt, red pepper flakes, and the remaining 6 tablespoons of olive oil and bring to boil. Reduce the heat to low, cover, and simmer for 15 to 60 minutes, allowing the flavors to blend. The longer the sauce cooks, the more flavorful it will be, but it will be ready to eat after 15 minutes of simmering.

3. Remove the sauce from the heat and stir in the basil. Serve warm. If not using right away, allow the sauce to cool to room temperature before storing in an airtight container in the refrigerator for up to four days.

Per Serving (1 cup): Calories: 226; Total Fat: 17g; Total Carbs: 19g; Net Carbs: 14g; Fiber: 5g; Protein: 4g; Sodium: 1036mg;
Macros: Fat: 68%, Carbs: 25%, Protein: 7%

OLIVE AND ARTICHOKE TAPENADE

Makes 2 cups | Prep Time: 10 minutes, plus 1 hour to marinate | Dairy-Free, Egg-Free, Gluten-Free, Nut-Free, Vegetarian

Tapenade is really just a fancy term for a spread or dip. Traditionally served with crackers or bread, this super flavorful condiment is great served with meat, fish, or scrambled eggs, or dolloped atop a fresh mixed greens salad. You can use green or black olives in this recipe, or try a combination of both!

- 1 cup finely chopped pitted Kalamata or Spanish Manzanilla olives
- 1 cup finely chopped artichoke hearts
- ¼ cup extra-virgin olive oil or avocado oil
- 2 teaspoons dried rosemary, oregano, parsley, basil, or thyme
- 1 garlic clove, minced
- ½ to 1 teaspoon red pepper flakes

1. In a medium bowl, combine the olives, artichoke hearts, olive oil, rosemary, garlic, and red pepper flakes and stir to combine. Marinate in the refrigerator, covered, for at least 1 hour before serving, to allow flavors to blend.

2. Store the tapenade in an airtight container in the refrigerator for up to one week.

VARIATION TIP: I love the chunky texture of this tapenade, but if you prefer a creamer texture, combine all the ingredients in a food processor and pulse until your desired consistency is reached.

Per Serving (¼ cup): Calories: 94; Total Fat: 9g; Total Carbs: 3g; Net Carbs: 0g; Fiber: 3g; Protein: 1g; Sodium: 332mg; **Macros:** Fat: 86%, Carbs: 10%, Protein: 4%

CREAMY LIME-CILANTRO DRESSING

Makes 1½ cups dressing | Prep Time: 10 minutes | Dairy-Free, Egg-Free, Gluten-Free, Nut-Free, Vegetarian

This creamy dressing is dairy-free and full of anti-inflammatory omega-3 fatty acids. It is wonderful as a ranch alternative on Cobb salads or drizzled over fajita bowls for added flavor.

- 2 very ripe avocados, pitted and peeled
- 1 cup packed fresh cilantro leaves
- ½ cup extra-virgin olive oil
- ¼ cup freshly squeezed lime juice (about 4 limes)
- 2 garlic cloves, peeled
- 1 teaspoon salt
- ½ teaspoon freshly ground black pepper

1. In a blender or tall wide container (if using an immersion blender), combine the avocados, cilantro, olive oil, lime juice, garlic, salt, and pepper and blend until thick and creamy. If the mixture seems too thick, add warm water, 1 tablespoon at a time.

2. Store the dressing in an airtight container in the refrigerator for up to one week.

Per Serving (2 tablespoons): Calories: 120; Total Fat: 13g; Total Carbs: 3g; Net Carbs: 1g; Fiber: 2g; Protein: 1g; Sodium: 199mg; **Macros:** Fat: 97%, Carbs: <1%, Protein: 3%

PERFECT RICED CAULIFLOWER

Serves 6 to 8 | Prep Time: 5 minutes | Cook Time: 10 minutes | Dairy-Free, Egg-Free, Gluten-Free, Nut-Free, Vegetarian

When chopped very finely, this versatile vegetable has the amazing ability to mimic the consistency of rice. While there are many commercially prepared versions nowadays, cauliflower has a high water content and most of these premade versions result in a mushy consistency when prepared to eat. Making your own is so easy, inexpensive, and flavor-preserving, I highly encourage you to give it a try.

1 small cauliflower head, broken into florets
¼ cup extra-virgin olive oil
2 garlic cloves, minced
2 teaspoons salt
½ to 1 teaspoon red pepper flakes
½ teaspoon ground turmeric (optional)
¼ to ½ cup chopped fresh basil, cilantro, or parsley

1. In a food processor, pulse the cauliflower several times, until it is the consistency of rice.

2. In a large skillet, heat the olive oil over medium-high heat. Add the cauliflower, garlic, salt, red pepper flakes, and turmeric (if using) and sauté for no more than 5 minutes.

3. Remove the cauliflower from the skillet and place in a large bowl to stop the cooking. Toss with the basil and serve warm.

Per Serving (½ cup): Calories: 93; Total Fat: 9g; Total Carbs: 3g; Net Carbs: 2g; Fiber: 1g; Protein: 1g; Sodium: 800mg;
Macros: Fat: 87%, Carbs: 9%, Protein: 4%

AVOCADO RANCH DRESSING

Makes about 2 cups | Prep Time: 10 minutes | Gluten-Free, Nut-Free, Vegetarian

Full of anti-inflammatory fats and void of pro-inflammatory ingredients, this dressing will be your new favorite! The avocado will naturally brown slightly as it is stored, so if you don't plan on using this all at once, I suggest halving the recipe. Although the color may change, the flavor will remain fresh and delicious.

- 1 very ripe avocado, pitted and peeled
- ½ cup Anti-Inflammatory Mayo (page 148)
- ½ cup full-fat buttermilk
- 2 tablespoons chopped fresh parsley, or 1 teaspoon dried parsley
- 2 tablespoons chopped red onion
- 1 tablespoon extra-virgin olive oil
- 1 tablespoon freshly squeezed lemon juice
- 2 teaspoons chopped fresh dill, or 1 teaspoon dried dill
- ½ teaspoon garlic powder
- ½ teaspoon salt
- ¼ teaspoon freshly ground black pepper

1. In a blender or tall wide container (if using an immersion blender), combine the avocado, mayo, buttermilk, parsley, onion, olive oil, lemon juice, dill, garlic powder, salt, and pepper and blend until thick and creamy, thinning out with additional lemon juice if necessary.

2. Store the dressing in an airtight container in the refrigerator for up to one week.

INGREDIENT TIP: If you don't have buttermilk on hand, combine ⅓ cup of heavy whipping cream with 1 tablespoon of fresh lemon juice and whisk until smooth.

Per Serving (2 tablespoons): Calories: 83; Total Fat: 9g; Total Carbs: 2g; Net Carbs: 1g; Fiber: 1g; Protein: 1g; Sodium: 122mg; **Macros:** Fat: 97%, Carbs: <1%, Protein: 3%

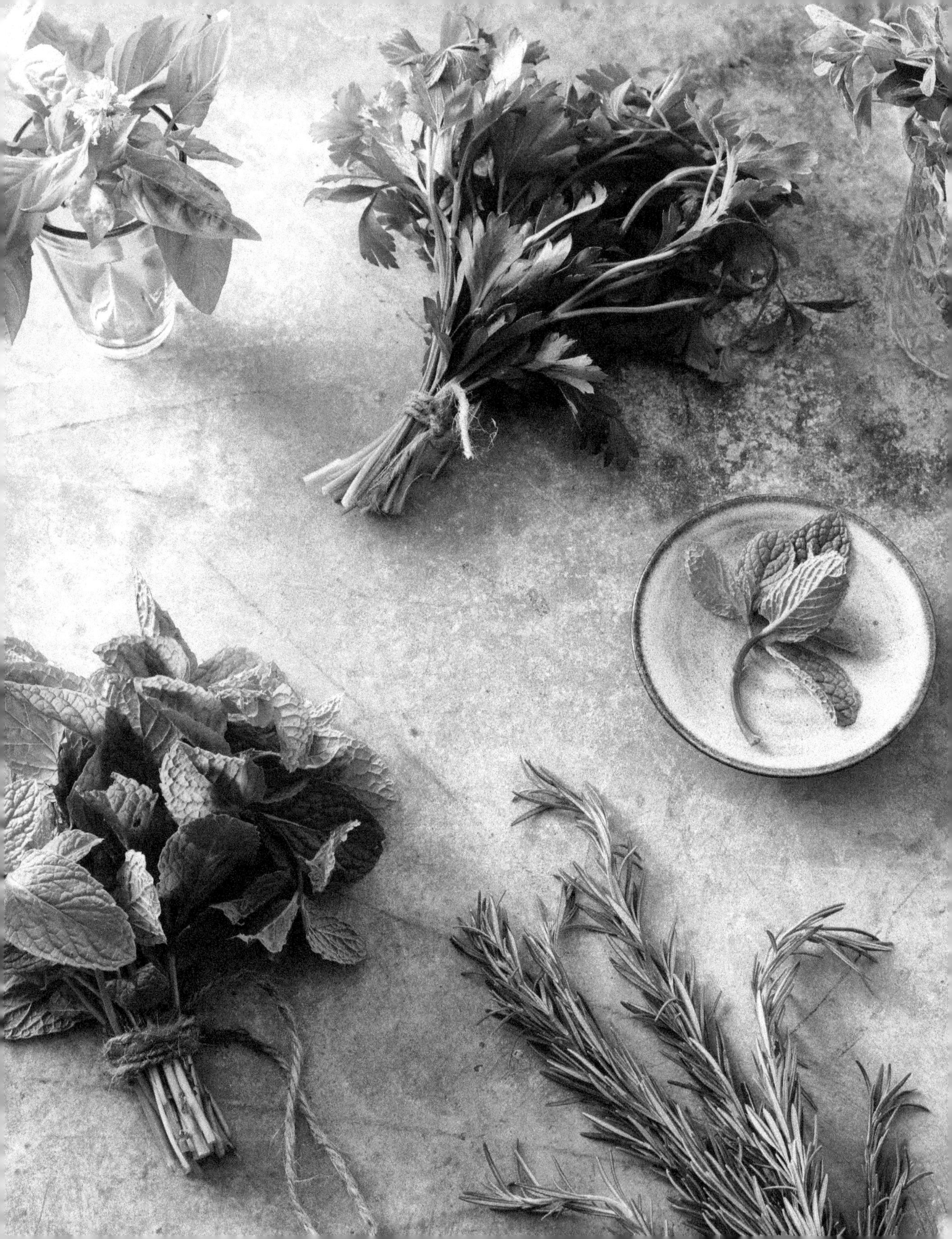

MEASUREMENT CONVERSIONS

Volume Equivalents (Liquid)

US STANDARD	US STANDARD (OUNCES)	METRIC (APPROXIMATE)
2 tablespoons	1 fl. oz.	30 mL
¼ cup	2 fl. oz.	60 mL
½ cup	4 fl. oz.	120 mL
1 cup	8 fl. oz.	240 mL
1½ cups	12 fl. oz.	355 mL
2 cups or 1 pint	16 fl. oz.	475 mL
4 cups or 1 quart	32 fl. oz.	1 L
1 gallon or 4 quarts	128 fl. oz.	4 L

Oven Temperatures

FAHRENHEIT	CELSIUS (APPROXIMATE)
250°F	120°C
300°F	150°C
325°F	165°C
350°F	180°C
375°F	190°C
400°F	200°C
425°F	220°C
450°F	230°C

Volume Equivalents (Dry)

US STANDARD	METRIC (APPROXIMATE)
⅛ teaspoon	0.5 mL
¼ teaspoon	1 mL
½ teaspoon	2 mL
¾ teaspoon	4 mL
1 teaspoon	5 mL
1 tablespoon	15 mL
¼ cup	59 mL
⅓ cup	79 mL
½ cup	118 mL
⅔ cup	156 mL
¾ cup	177 mL
1 cup	235 mL
2 cups or 1 pint	475 mL
3 cups	700 mL
4 cups or 1 quart	1 L

Weight Equivalents

US STANDARD	METRIC (APPROXIMATE)
½ ounce	15 g
1 ounce	30 g
2 ounces	60 g
4 ounces	115 g
8 ounces	225 g
12 ounces	340 g
16 ounces or 1 pound	455 g

REFERENCES

Aude, Y. W., Arthur S. Agatston, Francisco Lopez-Jimenez, Eric H. Lieberman, Marie Almon, Melinda Hansen, Gerardo Rojas, Gervasio A. Lamas, and Charles H. Hennekens. "The National Cholesterol Education Program Diet vs. a Diet Lower in Carbohydrates and Higher in Protein and Monounsaturated Fat: A Randomized Trial." *Archives of Internal Medicine* 164, no. 19 (October 2004): 2141–2146. doi:10.1001/archinte.164.19.2141.

Campos, H., J. J. Genest, Jr, E. Blijlevens, et al. "Low Density Lipoprotein Particle Size and Coronary Artery Disease." *Arteriosclerosis and Thrombosis: A Journal of Vascular Biology* 12, no. 2 (February 1992): 187–195. doi.org/10.1161/01.ATV.12.2.187.

Chung, H. Y., Dae Hyun Kim, Eun Kyeong Lee, Ki Wung Chung, et al. "Redefining Chronic Inflammation in Aging and Age-Related Diseases: Proposal of the Senoinflammation Concept." *Aging and Disease* 10, no. 2 (April 2019): 367–382. doi:10.14336/AD.2018.0324.

Dennis, E. A., and Paul C. Norris. "Eicosanoid Storm in Infection and Inflammation." *Nature Reviews Immuno*logy 15, no. 8 (August 2015): 511–523. doi:10.1038/nri3859.

de Sá Coutinho, D., Maria Talita Pacheco, Rudimar Luiz Frozza, and Andressa Bernardi. "Anti-Inflammatory Effects of Resveratrol: Mechanistic Insights." *International Journal of Molecular Science* 19, no. 6 (June 2018): 1812. doi:10.3390/ijms19061812.

Ellulu, M. S., Ismail Patimah, Huzwah Khaza'ai, Asmah Rahmat, and Yehia Abed. "Obesity and Inflammation: The Linking Mechanism and the Complications." *Archives of Medical Science* 13, no. 4 (June 2017): 851–863. doi:10.5114/aoms.2016.58928.

Foster, G. D., Holly Wyatt, James O. Hill, et al. "A Randomized Trial of a Low-Carbohydrate Diet for Obesity." *New England Journal of Medicine* 348, no. 21 (May 2003): 2082–2090. doi:10.1056/NEJMoa022207.

Freire, M. O., and Thomas E. Van Dyke. "Natural Resolution of Inflammation." *Periodontol 2000* 63, no. 1 (October 2013): 149–164. doi:10.1111/prd.12034.

Gardner, C. D., Alexandre Kiazand, Sofiya Alhassan, et al. "Comparison of the Atkins, Zone, Ornish, and LEARN Diets for Change in Weight and Related Risk Factors among Overweight Premenopausal Women." *Journal of the American Medical Association* 297, no. 9 (March 2007): 969–977. doi:10.1001/jama.297.9.969.

Haskó, G., and Bruce Cronstein. "Regulation of Inflammation by Adenosine." *Frontiers in Immuno*logy 4 (April 2013): 85. doi:10.3389/fimmu.2013.00085.

Kosinski, C., and F. R. Jornayvaz. "Effects of Ketogenic Diets on Cardiovascular Risk Factors: Evidence from Animal and Human Studies." *Nutrients* 9, no. 5 (May 2017): 517. doi:10.3390/nu9050517.

Kunnumakkara, A. B., Bethsebie L. Sailo, Kishore Banik, et al. "Chronic Diseases, Inflammation, and Spices: How Are They Linked?" *Journal of Translational Medicine* 16, no. 1 (2018): 14. doi:10.1186/s12967-018-1381-2.

Landry, A., Peter Docherty, Sylvie Ouellette, and Louis Jacques Cartier. "Causes and Outcomes of Markedly Elevated C-Reactive Protein Levels." *Canadian Family Physician* 63, no. 6 (June 2017): e316–e323.

Masino, Susan A., and David N. Ruskin. "Ketogenic Diets and Pain." *Journal of Child Neurology* 28, no. 8 (May 2013): 993–1001. doi:10.1177/0883073813487595.

Moon, Hyun-Seuk. "Chemopreventive Effects of Alpha Lipoic Acid on Obesity-Related Cancers." *Annals of Nutrition and Metabolism* 68, no. 2 (February 2016): 137–144. doi:10.1159/000443994.

Nagarkatti, P., Rupal Pandey, Sadiye Amcaoglu Rieder, Venkatesh L. Hegde, and Mitzi Nagarkatti. "Cannabinoids as Novel Anti-Inflammatory Drugs." *Future Medicinal Chemistry* 1, no. 7 (2009): 1333–1349. doi:10.4155/fmc.09.93.

Samaha, Frederick F., Nayyar Iqbal, Prakash Seshadri, et al. "A Low-Carbohydrate as Compared with a Low-Fat Diet in Severe Obesity." *New England Journal of Medicine* 348, no. 21 (May 2003): 2074–2081. doi:10.1056/NEJMoa022637.

Sproston N. R., and Jason J. Ashworth. "Role of C-Reactive Protein at Sites of Inflammation and Infection." *Frontiers in Immunology* 9 (April 2018): 754. doi:10.3389/fimmu.2018.00754.

Vidali, S., Sepideh Aminzadeh, Bridget Lambert, et al. "Mitochondria: The Ketogenic Diet: A Metabolism-Based Therapy." *International Journal of Biochemistry and Cell Biology* 63 (June 2015): 55–59. doi:10.1016/j.biocel.2015.01.022.

Weisenberger, Jill. "The Omega Fats." *Today's Dietitian* 16, no. 4 (2014): 20. https://www.todaysdietitian.com/newarchives/040114p20.shtml.

Wood, Richard J., Jeff Volek, Yanzhu Liu, et al. "Carbohydrate Restriction Alters Lipoprotein Metabolism by Modifying VLDL, LDL, and HDL Subfraction Distribution and Size in Overweight Men." *The Journal of Nutrition* 136, no. 2 (February 2006): 384–389. doi.org/10.1093/jn/136.2.384.

INDEX

C

D

E

H

I

K

L

M

N

O

P

R

S

W

Y

Z

ACKNOWLEDGMENTS

This project was written during a global pandemic. What we will surely all one day refer to as "The Year of COVID-19," 2020 has certainly had its challenges. One silver lining I have found, and encourage my clients to also find, is the pause from our hurried chaotic lifestyles and the necessity to revert back to a "simpler" time of home-cooked meals, more time with family (for better or for worse!), and the ability to make time to focus on self-care. In an uncertain time when so much is out of our control, the one thing we *can* control is doing our best to improve our health and nutrition.

As always, I am grateful for my amazing patients and clients; you are the reason I do what I do and do it with such passion. My family: Brent, Harper, Luke, Evan, Geege, Dats, Jean, Matt, Louise, and Hattie. Feeding you makes my heart full. For all of my foodie friends who always inspire me in every way: I hope to cook with you again soon!

I also want to thank the fantastic team at Callisto Media who make the writing process seamless and fun. I am so happy to have you by my side.

ABOUT THE AUTHOR

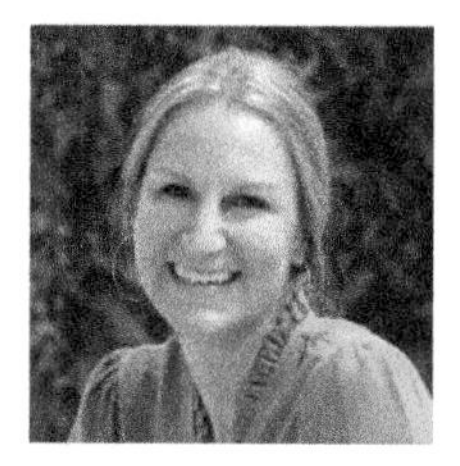

Molly Devine is a registered dietitian who specializes in digestive health, healthy weight management, and chronic disease prevention through integrative and functional nutrition. She is an advocate for sustainable lifestyle change through nutrition intervention and the founder of MSD Nutrition Consulting and Eat Your Keto, a nutrition counseling and individualized meal planning service focusing on customized whole foods–based diets for disease prevention and management. She utilizes telehealth to work with clients across the country.

Molly is the author of *Essential Ketogenic Mediterranean Diet Cookbook: 100 Low-Carb, Heart-Healthy Recipes for Lasting Weight Loss* and *The Natural Candida Cleanse: A Healthy Treatment Guide to Improve Your Microbiome*; the coauthor of *The Ketogenic Lifestyle: How to Fuel Your Best*; and a regular contributor to nutrition-based online media such as *Shape*, *Insider*, *Greatist*, *HuffPost*, *Brides*, and ABC11 *Eyewitness News*.

Molly received her bachelor of science in nutrition sciences from North Carolina Central University and completed her dietetic internship through Meredith College. She also holds a bachelor of science in languages and linguistics from Georgetown University. She lives in Durham, North Carolina, with her family.

CPSIA information can be obtained
at www.ICGtesting.com
Printed in the USA
JSHW030402301121
20827JS00003B/6